34 Patients

34 Patients

*What Becoming a Doctor Taught Me About
Health, Hope and Humanity*

TOM TEMPLETON

MICHAEL 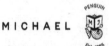 JOSEPH

MICHAEL JOSEPH

UK | USA | Canada | Ireland | Australia
India | New Zealand | South Africa

Michael Joseph is part of the Penguin Random House group of companies
whose addresses can be found at global.penguinrandomhouse.com

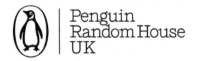

First published 2021

001

Copyright © Tom Templeton, 2021

The moral right of the author has been asserted

This book is substantially a work of non-fiction based on the life, experiences and recollections of the author.
To maintain patient confidentiality and to protect the privacy of individuals, names of people/places/dates/
sequences of the detail of events have been changed and certain situations and individuals may
have been merged to further protect identities. Any similarities are purely coincidental.

Set in 13.5/16pt Garamond MT Std
Typeset by Jouve (UK), Milton Keynes
Printed and bound in Great Britain by Clays Ltd, Elcograf S.p.A.

The authorized representative in the EEA is Penguin Random House Ireland,
Morrison Chambers, 32 Nassau Street, Dublin D02 YH68

A CIP catalogue record for this book is available from the British Library

HARDBACK ISBN: 978-0-241-42933-4
TRADE PAPERBACK ISBN: 978-0-241-42934-1

www.greenpenguin.co.uk

For Siobhán, Oscar, Molly and Sam

Life is short.
Hippocrates

Life is long.
Seneca

Life is what happens to you while
you're busy making other plans.
John Lennon

Contents

Prologue

Perhaps you're on the bus looking across the aisle at a scruffy woman with purple hair jerking her head up to the ceiling. What's wrong with her? Why does she keep muttering to herself?

How about the middle-aged man in the suit playing *Candy Crush* on his phone? He had a heart attack two months ago and now he's worried every twinge in his chest is a sign of impending death. He can't concentrate at work or at home, his marriage is on the rocks, all because he feels unbearably vulnerable all the time. The phone game is a brief attempt to escape.

The mum ignoring the screaming child is worried sick about how she'll cope without *her* mum, who has just been diagnosed with ovarian cancer. The grumpy-looking old woman with the annoying shopping trolley just left her demented husband with the carer and has multiple chores to do in the precious hour before she has to get back. She's increasingly forgetful because of the stress, and is worried she might be losing her marbles too. That guy with the hipster beard, nodding happily along to whatever's blaring out on his headphones, found a lump on his testicle a few months ago but he's too scared to see the doctor. He'll be relieved when he goes eventually and is told it's benign. Several other passengers are on their way to hospital or doctors' appointments. Why is the bus driver driving so slowly? She is preoccupied with memories of her young nephew who died on this day ten years ago.

Everyone you see on this bus today has lost a loved one.

And what about you? What are you carrying with you? Do you sometimes rub that arm you broke as a child and feel the lump it left behind? Is your older brother still under section on the mental health ward? Have you had a double mastectomy? Did you contemplate suicide some years back? Is your already stressful life becoming overwhelming with the Covid-19 pandemic? You've also spent time in the borderlands between sickness and health, and you too carry the scars.

Looking back at the muttering woman, maybe she isn't as odd as you first thought. Maybe we're all odd, all suffering, all normal. Look out of the window. It's raining. Or is it sunny? It's incredible to be alive. Damn it, the doors have opened and it's your stop. Quick! Get up, get out and get on with your life.

In 1999, aged eighteen, I had a summer-holiday job as a ward clerk at St Thomas' Hospital in London. I'd been placed there by a temp agency and had no interest in medicine at the time. The work itself felt routine, banal. In a high-ceilinged Victorian ward overlooking the River Thames I logged patients on to the computer system, chased down medical notes and X-rays in the far reaches of the hospital and made many cups of tea for the nurses. But although I hadn't especially wanted to work there and was doing it to help fund the next year of university, the hospital quickly became a profound environment for me. The patients were what changed things. They came from all parts of society, from rough sleepers to aristocrats. Some were dying rapidly, some were temporarily ill, others chronically so. Some shouted and sobbed, while some did everything to avoid emotion. I didn't understand much of what was going on, but I could see how vital it was, and how different it was to what I saw in my everyday life.

I was particularly struck by one patient. Others were in and out (or had died) within days or weeks but Jack was bedded in, and seemed as if he'd always been there. A few months earlier he had gone for a drink with his partner. They'd chosen an old haunt, the Admiral Duncan, a popular gay pub in Soho. Though they didn't know it as they went in chatting, another young man had left his sports bag by the bar. While Jack was queuing for a drink the rudimentary explosives in the bag were detonated by a cheap alarm clock. Packed around them were 500 nails. Three people, including a pregnant woman and her unborn child, were killed.

'Seventy wounded,' said the papers the next day. At St Thomas' I got a small taste of what 'wounded' meant for one person. I saw nothing of the on-scene and subsequent hospital efforts to prevent Jack bleeding to death from his stump. I didn't witness the touch-and-go month in intensive care, the several revision surgeries that followed. Two months after the bomb blast, what I saw was a man with scars on his arms and a colostomy bag, whose leg ended just below the knee, awkwardly navigating the hospital ward in a wheelchair or on crutches.

Jack and I used to chat about football. He lived for visits from friends and family; his spirits always plummeted when they left. As I got to know him I discovered this wasn't the first hurdle in his life. He told me that, years before the bombing, he'd suffered from depression and alcohol dependence.

Now he was learning to walk again, struggling with severe pain, deafness and post-traumatic stress disorder. Struggling to make sense of the vicious act that had occurred and its consequences for him. 'Why,' he used to ask, 'why did this happen to me?'

The perpetrator was caught the day after the bombing and placed in a different sort of institution – a hospital for mentally ill prisoners. He was diagnosed with paranoid schizophrenia and a possible personality disorder before being transferred to prison years later.

Until that summer I had always thought of the NHS as a bland, antiseptic institution. Up till then it had meant the drab waiting room at the local GP surgery I scarcely visited. This holiday job opened my eyes to what I now know is the reality. The hospitals and surgeries of this country are a pulsating, variegated hive of pain, lunacy, death, sorrow, redemption and recovery, and when a stone crashes into the waters of a life many of the ripples wash on to its shores.

After two months I went off to university and left Jack still on the ward. Later I became a newspaper journalist. My dream job. We reported the news and moved on. I loved the breadth of what we covered, and the speed of it, the lofty heights from which we operated. Naturally much of what we reported on was human suffering. And as the stones began to fall in my life – a friend who had a psychotic breakdown, an aunt who died of ovarian cancer – I began to find the distance between the lofty heights and that suffering uncomfortable.

One day I was walking down the street to lunch when I glanced down an alleyway and saw a paramedic trying to resuscitate a dead man. A shocking sight – not least *because* of how shocking it was, despite happening every day in this city. After that I found myself thinking more and more often about Jack with his stump and his crutches searching for meaning in the borderlands.* I began wondering if the answer to all this suffering could be found back where my holiday job had briefly taken me, in medicine.

When I walked into the medical school lecture theatre, aged thirty, I became immersed in an expanding wealth of knowledge about the way the body worked. The names and inner workings of disease after disease, the symptoms they cause, the risk factors for them, the investigations and treatments, the likely outcomes. We covered the causes and effects of hundreds of illnesses at the molecular, microscopic, naked-eye, statistical, psychological, cultural, political and societal levels.

The ocean of suffering that medicine deals with expanded for me and came into sharper focus. Like many of my colleagues I occasionally suffered from 'medical student syndrome', where I would begin to believe, with greater or lesser irrationality, that I was suffering from the symptoms of an illness that we had recently been taught about. I also became more realistic about the limitations of our knowledge and our treatments, and of the scale of the struggle to advance medicine in the lab.

As I left the lecture theatre for the wards, grand ideas of saving lives gave way to fears that I would screw up and end them. The limitations of medicine stopped being theoretical. We generally do our best with what we have but it is often not enough. In your first years practising as a doctor you

* Jack has since died.

spend time working in many different specialties in order to gain broad experience before deciding which area to specialize in. As I moved from psychiatry to orthopaedics, from intensive care to general practice, from A & E to internal medicine, from geriatrics to paediatrics, the excitement of the work was always tempered by the sorrow and distress I witnessed. Even in cases where we 'cured' the patient I could see their time in the borderlands left them with a new emotional scar. An invisible tattoo. But this was real life, I thought, why is it that we so often deny it and edit it out?

In the past decade of training and working I've had the privilege of meeting thousands of patients from different walks and stages of life and from different cultures. Patients who have suffered every imaginable kind of physical and psychological trauma. Doctors are the priests of our society; patients bare their souls as well as their bodies. The stories of these thirty-four patients, from a stillborn child to a 103-year-old woman, draw back the curtain on life spent in these borderlands: men, women and children struggling against the reality of bodily betrayal, psychological fragility and social deprivation, and medicine's inadequate efforts to rectify this.

I've written them down because even if the medicine didn't always heal, the capacity for humans to understand, to endure and to love seemed to provide some sort of redemption. The borderlands can be a frightening place, but an unflinching look at life there is cathartic. It seems to me that we hide these segments of our lives at our peril. We can learn from our suffering and the suffering of others, and use it to help us understand our lives better and to reorient ourselves.

Facing the fragility of human existence should help us to celebrate it.

Author's Note

34 Patients tells the stories inspired by patients I encountered while training and working as a doctor. The stories are told in chronological order of the patient's age, from the youngest to the oldest. As a result the locations and my age and level of medical experience moves backwards and forwards throughout the book.

The names and other identifying details of all patients, relatives and colleagues have been changed to maintain patient confidentiality and ensure that no one will recognize loved ones or even themselves. Certain situations and individuals may have been merged to further protect identities. Any resemblance to persons living or dead that has occurred as a result of these changes will be by coincidence.

At the end of the book are notes on the diseases suffered by these patients.

Childhood

Snow in May

It's May and there is a blizzard in town. We walk shivering in navy scrubs across the courtyard, snowflakes circling softly down to earth, muffling the shrieks and cries of the city. On the far side we enter a low-slung grey breeze-block building. We both show an ID card to a pale man, spectacles propped up on a nose crackling with red blood vessels. We explain why we've come and he stands up with a sigh and leads us into a cold room, unlocks a freezer door and pulls out a sliding metal tray. On it is a plastic crate the size of a shoebox. He opens the lid and inside is a dead baby wrapped in muslin. Its ears are remarkably tiny and low slung, its forehead is bulging, its eyes too widely spaced.

We look at it for ten seconds, which feels like an eternity. I think of how the baby lived for thirty-nine weeks in the womb but never got to see the outside world. I think of the stuffed toy monkey that lay waiting in the cot throughout the labour. The parents already back in their empty home.

Too quickly the man closes the lid, pushes the tray in and closes the freezer door on the baby. We walk out into a warmer room, still shivering as we sit down, and are given a book in which my colleague writes in black ink. He writes the date, the names of the parents, his own name and medical registration and a cause of death: congenital abnormality.

The baby also has a name, which is written.

The man takes the book from my colleague. We walk back

through the two pairs of doors and out into the thickening snow, which obscures the hospital from us. Cold as it is I don't want to reach the hospital on the other side of the courtyard with its rooms full of mothers giving birth.

'Snow in May,' my colleague says, squinting up at the sky, and shakes his head.

Rap Birth

After thirty-six hours the screaming stops and there is silence from the people in the room and everyone is still. My neonatology colleague and I have just arrived in response to a bleep.

It is a small room in the delivery ward, dark apart from a low orange spotlamp illuminating a tableau, like a festive nativity scene. The people in the scene cast long shadows. The young woman is on her back in a baggy T-shirt, legs up in stirrups, and between her legs is a tiny purple face, heavy jowls smeared with white vernix. Eyes closed. Not crying. Not breathing. Body still inside its mother. On the cusp.

To the woman's right is a friend, smartly dressed and heavily made-up for the occasion. She can see the baby's head and is wiping away tears of joy and relief. She clutches a soft toy lion. To the woman's left, holding her hand, is the midwife, elfin in bright green scrubs. Behind her, in a purple smock, is her assistant, two years in the country, sending most of her pay cheque back to three young children left behind in the Philippines.

Sitting on a stool between the mother's legs is the obstetrician dressed in navy scrubs. The baby's heart rate had been worryingly slow for a few hours, so before the last set of contractions she attached a suction cup to its head, made a snip to the woman's perineum with some shears and pulled on the cup in time with the contractions to assist the head's passage into the world. The cup has now been removed.

The slow heart rate is why we were bleeped and why we now stand in the corner of the small room round an incubator, its red warming lamp switched on, suction and breathing gear ready just in case the baby, once born, needs help surviving.

The woman sucks down laughing gas through a plastic tube. The legend on her T-shirt says EVERYBODY DIES BUT NOT EVERYBODY LIVES.

A quick glance at her medical notes shows she is seventeen years old, and a first-time mother. She has mental health problems. The baby's father has drug dependencies and 'is not involved'. Medical details. Everything else left out.

'I'll put on the song you chose,' her friend says, 'for the birth,' and presses buttons on a phone.

Now a rap song emerges tinnily into the quiet of the room.

> *When the stars shine bright*
> *They scare me to death*
> *I light up the pipe*
> *Just to give me some breath*

'So with the next contractions I want you to push really hard,' says the obstetrician.

'I can't,' says the mother. 'I can't do it.'

'You're doing so well,' says the obstetrician. 'And this is the last time, I promise. And then your baby will be born.'

The midwife chips in, trying to keep it casual. 'Would you like me to put the baby on your chest when he comes out?'

There's a long pause.

'Not right away,' the mother says.

I glance at the mother's face. It is drawn, pale, beaded with sweat.

Then the midwife, almost pleading, says, 'I'll hold him and we'll clean him; it'll be good for you to be close straight away.'

The mother takes another inhalation of the laughing gas. A single tear rolls from her right eye. 'I don't want him straight away,' she says.

'I'll help,' says her friend. 'You'll be fine.'

'I can't,' she says. 'I don't want him.'

There is silence from the people in the room. Everyone is still. The baby's not yet born face impassive in the orange light.

> *The motherfucking jeep*
> *Don't start the first time*
> *I can't get to sleep*
> *Case it's for the last time*
> *You're bringing the bills*
> *I'm bringing the dope*
> *They're bringing their guns*
> *Now we just gotta hope*

'They're coming,' screams the mother.

'OK, push deep with the contractions,' says the midwife, gripping her hand tight.

'You can do it,' says her friend.

'Come on,' says the Filipino healthcare assistant.

The mother is wailing and moaning, trying to suck on the laughing gas, but in too much pain to get the tube to her mouth.

'Keep pushing,' says the obstetrician, gripping the baby by the neck and twisting to release first one shoulder, and then, after what seems like an age – what with the mother's screaming, and everyone else holding their breath – the other shoulder comes and the whole baby slithers out while the rest of the amniotic fluid splatters on to the floor. The baby is swung up to the midwife, who wraps and rubs him with a towel next to the mother, who looks away, exhausted. Her friend cries, everyone else smiles involuntarily, and there is more silence.

Don't care 'bout the army they send
We fight together
I got your back, right to the end
Don't care 'bout the army they send
We fight together
Me and you blazin', right to the end

The baby is wrapped in a new towel, a white cotton hat put on his head. He cries heartily, an excellent sign. We start packing up the resuscitation gear and turn off the red warming lamp.

'Do you want to feed him?' asks the midwife.

The mother shakes her head almost imperceptibly. She is still facing towards her friend, in our direction, resolutely looking away from the baby held by the midwife on the far side of the bed. Her friend strokes the mother's pale, drawn face.

'He's gorgeous,' she says gently.

The mother pushes the friend's hand away and takes another drag of the laughing gas. The healthcare assistant takes the swaddled baby from the midwife, offers him a bottle of formula milk, ready prepared and warmed. The baby hungrily grabs at the rubber teat with his mouth and starts sucking. His umbilical cord stretches down and into his mother, legs still up in the stirrups, still sucking away on the gas and air.

The friend offers the toy lion to the mother. 'Why don't you give this to him?' she asks.

The mother shakes her head. Despite all these people crammed into the room around her she looks completely alone. There is another silence.

'He's so beautiful,' says the purple-clad healthcare assistant, making it all look so easy as she feeds the baby. In a studiedly neutral voice she asks the mother a question. 'Did you decide in the end what you wanted to call him?'

I look over at the mother and suddenly I feel my heart pounding in my chest. She pauses with the gas and air nozzle at her mouth, her pale young face taut with fear. She looks paralysed. Then she turns her head to face forward for the first time, still not looking at the baby, but not looking away.

'He's called Noah,' she says.

The mother inhales the room's air deeply, looking fiercely at the orange spotlamp.

The healthcare assistant moves a little closer to her with the baby.

The obstetrician clamps and then snips the umbilical cord.

My colleague and I leave, not needed now to help the baby.

Hunger

The shouts and cries from the corridor get louder as Johnny approaches. I can make out a child's voice. 'Gim bic, gim bic,' it seems to be saying, then degenerates into a howl.

There's a final roar and a large buggy arrives in the door frame of the consultation room. The boy in the buggy is arching his back in fury and the glittering gold baseball cap on his head gets pushed forward so it covers his eyes. This enrages him so much that he grabs the hat from his head and bites the brim.

At this moment he notices a strange adult looming over him. He pauses chubby-faced, hat gripped in his mouth, baby-blue eyes flickering from me to the computer, the couch, the window, then back to me again. As if deciding I am no great threat, he roars again and hurls the golden cap across the room.

Leaning on the back of the buggy, apologizing profusely for being late is his father, Wayne. He is tubby, sweating and clutching a silver knapsack. I pick the gold cap off the floor and Johnny's dad hangs it on one buggy handle, then hangs his silver bag on the other. They dangle there like resting planets.

Wayne manoeuvres his way round the buggy, unstraps Johnny, muttering soothing chitchat to him – 'Here we are, Johnny. Here we are.' – and hauls him with difficulty out of the chair.

Johnny is noticeably overweight, far larger than you would think he'd had time to become in his three and a half years; he looks more than four stone. He is briefly held by his father in a standing position and his legs bow as if scarcely able to take his weight before he plops him down on the lino floor. Johnny immediately reaches up, arms wide open in supplication, like a felled striker appealing for a penalty or a wronged worshipper appealing to their god. He makes beseeching, mewling cries at his father.

Wayne looks at his son. 'No, Johnny,' he says. 'I'm not giving you anything.'

He heads to the chair by my desk. Johnny's cries turn to ear-splitting roars, the word 'dadda' emerging from the wall of noise. He shuffles on his bottom towards Wayne and starts bouncing his bulk up and down in a demonstration of fury.

Wayne is hovering above his seat. He looks at me, then guiltily away, stands back up and rifles through the silver knapsack. Johnny goes silent, his pale blue eyes watching his father like a hawk. Wayne's hands emerge from the bag holding biscuits. Now Johnny is bouncing with excitement. He snatches the biscuits and begins guzzling, with sounds of pleasure.

Wayne slumps in the chair by my desk and sits back in it with a sigh of fatigue. He looks exhausted, dwarfed by the room. Momentarily tears spring to his eyes.

'Are you OK?' I ask.

He nods, unable to speak, and quickly erases the tears with the heel of his hand. His face is young, surely early twenties at most, he has shaved but missed a patch on his neck which shows red stubble. He has intelligent, watchful eyes, a gold stud in one ear and brand new trainers, daunting in their pristine whiteness, like a field of freshly fallen snow.

Johnny sits on the floor, the stub of the first biscuit in his mouth, jowls covered in saliva and wet biscuit remnants, the second biscuit clutched in his right hand. His milky-white belly is bursting out of a bright red jumper embossed with the phrase SUGAR DADDY and stretching the elastic waistband of his denim jeans.

He looks at me with a mixture of triumph and suspicion. I stare back.

'Tell me why you're here,' I say.

Wayne takes a deep breath and launches into their story.

Johnny was born at term a healthy weight and size. Wayne's partner found the idea of breastfeeding unpleasant, so it was straight on to the bottle, but a few days after they got him home he was struggling to suckle the teat properly and he lost a lot of weight. Back in hospital he was fed through a tube passed into his nose and down into his stomach while the doctors tried to work out what was going on. After ruling out the more common things, they did genetic testing and found Johnny had a rare condition called Prader–Willi syndrome. Johnny was five days old when his mother and father were called into a little room and given the diagnosis and told that this condition was incurable.

'Michelle burst into tears,' Wayne says, 'I just felt unable to move, as if I had no strength. It took us a while to get it together.'

'I'm not surprised,' I say.

'The doctor said it was normal for people to go into shock when they get the news, but –' he shakes his head – 'I'm not sure Chelle ever got over it.'

'Where is she?' I ask.

A cloud crosses his face. 'She died,' he says. 'Cancer.'

'I'm sorry,' I say, 'How long ago?'

'Year and a half.' His face is tense as he mentions her.

'How are you doing with all of that?' I ask.

'I'm OK. I've got Johnny,' he says, looking with pleasure at his son. 'We're OK aren't we, Johnny?'

Johnny is on to his second biscuit and doesn't seem to care.

'Problem is everything else the doctors said turned out true.'

'Such as?'

'They said Johnny would need help feeding at first because he hadn't got the muscles to do it himself, but once he's big enough to feed himself he'll be starvin' hungry all the time and there'll be no stopping him. And they told me it's my job to keep him from getting fat, to stop him from eating himself sick. And now look,' he says, pointing at Johnny. He shakes his head bitterly in disgust at himself. 'I feel like I can't do anything right.'

Johnny has finished the biscuits and is licking his crumb-coated fists. He stares at me with open curiosity and suspicion. I stare back. Not only has he lost his mother but the genetic test has read Johnny's chemical stars. We all know things about kids' futures that they don't, but it feels particularly dreadful to see Johnny's destiny this clearly.

Somewhere in the intricate microscopic dance of Johnny's genes a misstep has taken place. Now an almond-sized gland in his brain, a few centimetres behind his eyes, is pumping out chemicals that are giving him the stomach-gnawing, un-ignorable sensation of hunger until he has eaten five times as many calories as he needs. Five bananas instead of one. Ten biscuits instead of two. Fifteen fish fingers instead of three. From the moment he wakes until the moment he falls asleep he will feel the magnificently evolved, sledgehammer craving of hunger. He is destined to be ravenous for his whole life.

Johnny sits on his bottom with legs curled in front of him like crab claws. They look floppy with the feet oddly curved down at the ankle. People with Prader–Willi syndrome have slower metabolisms and weaker muscles – hence the difficulty suckling when new born. Put these things together and the deck is heavily stacked towards life-shortening obesity. Then there are problems with behaviour, intellect, fertility.

Johnny is beginning to bounce on his haunches again, supplicating for food.

'Gim bic,' he says to his father. 'Gim bic.'

'No, Johnny, you don't need a biscuit,' Wayne says.

To try to distract him I grab a box of toys and bring it over.

Johnny frowns and beckons towards them. I fake a frown back at him. Then I suddenly smile. Johnny looks taken aback, then smiles himself.

There is a wooden farm with animals. I hold out a small duck in my hand. To get to it he shuffles towards me on his bottom. He snatches at it but I pull it away and close it in my fist.

He looks at me uncertainly. I offer him my closed fist then open it. There's the duck. He laughs. Now I switch the duck back and forth rapidly between my hands and offer him two closed fists. He gets the idea and stares at the fists. Then touches one of them. Finger by finger I reveal an empty palm. He looks up at me and quickly touches the other fist, and finger by finger I reveal the duck. He laughs with pleasure and takes the duck from me then pops it into his mouth for safekeeping.

Now he wants the bull. I play at withholding that for a while then let him take it.

He gets interested in the wooden creatures so I turn back to Wayne. But then I notice Johnny holding out a fist to me, bull clearly sticking out of it.

I can't help but laugh and take it from him.

He grins at me.

'Moooo,' I say, waggling the bull.

He pulls the duck out of his mouth. 'Wha,' he says.

'So Johnny is three and a half now,' I say. 'How are you guys getting on?'

Wayne breathes in deeply as if this is a test he needs to pass. 'Johnny's doing really well. Aren't you, Johnny?'

Johnny seems oblivious, clapping like a seal and wiggling his legs, a toy animal in each hand. Happily the centre of his universe.

'We sing songs, go to the park, watch TV together, eat together. Johnny doesn't sleep well so we sleep in the same bed, which is fine but he wakes me up early, hungry.'

'Do you have anyone else to help out?' I ask.

Wayne winces. 'I'm not in contact with my family,' he says. 'We fell out. They didn't like Chelle and cut us out. When she died . . . I can't forgive them. I don't want them around Johnny . . .' He tails off.

This is obviously not a comfortable subject.

'Chelle's mum is down in Cornwall – we see her twice a year. I've lost touch with my friends; the ones who have kids don't really understand Johnny's condition and how difficult he can be, so we can't do the things they want to do. And the ones who don't have kids . . .' he grins. 'Well, obviously they don't understand.'

'Nursery?'

'Not yet.'

'So every day it's just you two at home?' I ask, struggling to imagine what this must be like.

He nods.

'It doesn't sound as if you get any time to yourself,' I say.

Tears hover in his eyes again and I push the box of tissues to Wayne's end of the desk.

'I'm sorry,' he says, dabbing at his eyes. 'I love him but it's hard.'

'Totally understandable,' I say.

'He's great,' says Wayne, 'until he loses his temper, and then he really loses it. He chucks himself backwards. I'm afraid he's going to hurt himself one day, and I'm worried I'm not going to be able to pick him up soon.'

We look at Johnny who is trying to give me the wooden bull.

I cover my eyes in fear and Johnny bellows at the bull telling it off for frightening me and drops it down the chimney of a plastic doll's house.

'Is he standing at all?' I ask. 'Walking?'

'With help,' Wayne says.

I stand up, and hold my hands out to Johnny to see what he can do. He grabs my hands and I feel his trusting grip. I pull him upwards gently and he responds by putting some tension in his legs and digging his heels into the carpet and soon he is standing. He is taking the weight on his legs but they bow a little. We manage a few steps of a sort of shambolic dance before his legs give way, I grab him around the side and we manage an ungraceful sit back down. In that assisted fall I feel his full weight. Wayne looks on, concerned. If Johnny doesn't lose some weight or learn to walk soon, he may never manage.

I offer him my hands again and, game, despite the fall, he stands and allows himself to be guided to the weighing scales with a seat attached. When he slumps down into it we see he weighs thirty-one kilograms. Plotted against the standard lines on the growth chart Johnny's weight is taking off like a rocket. He is heavy for a boy double his age.

'I don't know how he's putting on so much weight,' says Wayne. 'I don't feed him more than the dieticians said I should. But if I don't watch carefully, he'll snatch food from my plate. We were in a caff the other day and he leaned over and stole this old woman's toast off her plate. She told me I should be ashamed, bringing up a child so bad. I gave her a piece of my mind. I don't care that they see a fat useless dad but when they see a fat useless boy it . . . it makes me want to kill them.'

I nod in sympathy.

'I'm trying,' he says, 'I'm really trying, but it's hard to leave him hungry. I just want him to be happy.'

'This was always going to be the big challenge,' I say.

'Anyway,' he says, 'the reason I'm here is to see if there really is a cure.'

I'm taken aback. 'A cure?'

'Yeah, I've been reading on the internet something about a pill that would stop Johnny being hungry.'

Noticing the lack of affirmation on my face Wayne looks wounded. 'I know you can't believe everything you see on the internet,' he adds quietly.

I'm pretty sure that there is no cure. This is one of those illnesses where an almost superhuman amount of effort and discipline is required from everyone involved simply to reduce the inevitable damage. That and a perspective change about what Johnny's life can involve. But I don't want to slam the door in Wayne's face.

'I'm not aware of a cure,' I say, 'but let's look it up.'

We huddle round the computer and I search for recent papers on treatments. Predictably there are several anti-hunger medications being trialled but nothing proven effective or safe enough to use.

'I'm sorry,' I say, 'I'm sure the hospital doctors will let you know if anything new becomes available. In the meantime we have to help you with everything else in Johnny's life: dieticians, physios, education.'

Wayne starts sobbing silently to himself, shoulders shuddering. When he regains control he says, 'It's the hope that kills me. I can't stop thinking one day there'll be a pill that will change everything.'

Johnny notices his father's tears. With great effort he shuffles towards him and grabs his legs as if to comfort him.

'It's OK, Johnny,' Wayne says, wiping his eyes with his sleeve. 'I'm OK.'

Knowing he cannot pick him up he gets down on the floor to give him a cuddle. Johnny lays his head on Wayne's chest and allows himself to be swallowed up in his embrace.

'I'm sorry,' Wayne says from the floor, Johnny in his arms. 'Nothing in my life seems to go right.'

And then it comes: the drunken father, bullied mother, leaving home as a teenager to move in with a girlfriend who then cheated on him, his job at the printworks, becoming supervisor after a few years, then the shoulder injury that finished that job, then the depression that followed, then meeting Michelle and their blazing romance, and then Johnny. And then the cancer taking Michelle away.

'He's the best thing in my life,' Wayne says simply. 'I couldn't have asked for better.'

I look at Wayne now as if seeing him for the first time. Tubby, sweating, partially shaven face strained with desperation. Hoping for a pill. Asked by doctors in their tidy offices to withhold food from his only child.

'Is there anything else I can help with?' I ask.

He hesitates and then looks away. 'There is actually,' he says, staring at the wall. 'I'm . . . There's a woman I've started seeing and . . . well, it's not serious at the moment, but I wanted to know . . .' He carefully places his hands over Johnny's ears then turns and looks up at me with his young pale face. 'Well, if I was ever to have another kid . . . would they come out like Johnny?'

I shake my head. 'There is almost no possibility of that happening,' I say. 'Johnny having this was a bolt of lightning, complete . . . chance.'

Johnny struggles out of Wayne's grasp and shuffles over to the buggy and starts rooting around in the silver knapsack, presumably looking for some food. Wayne gets up and lifts the bag out of reach. Johnny is enraged. He lets out a wail and strikes at his father, but his aim is poor. Frustrated he throws himself back on to the lino of the consulting room and howls at the ceiling, flailing his four limbs about. He is inconsolable.

As Wayne hauls him into the pushchair Johnny suddenly goes limp. He has stopped crying, stopped shouting. Wayne gently lets go of him. Johnny looks at me, then he bottom-shuffles across the floor and snatches the wooden bull from the chimney of the doll's house.

Staring up at me with his pale blue eyes, he shuffles across the floor towards me and hands me the toy. 'Boo,' he says.

'Thank you,' I say. We smile at each other.

Wayne manhandles him into the buggy and clicks the belt shut. The golden baseball cap is put on Johnny's head then hurled across the room, then retrieved and thrust into the bag. Throughout his endeavours I notice a tattoo on Wayne's forearm with the word *Michelle* and two dates. Johnny starts roaring again as they exit the room.

I watch them walk down the corridor and past a waiting room full of patients, several of whom stare in open disgust at Johnny and his dad. One woman tuts and shakes her head. Johnny's roaring recedes as the electric surgery doors slide open and let them both out into the sun. One to a lifetime of hunger and the other to a lifetime of keeping him hungry.

Oxygen

The small blonde girl is struggling to breathe by the time she arrives at the emergency department. We can see that in the shallow movements of her chest, the way her neck muscles tug with each breath and by the panic written across her face.

I can also see fear in the eyes of her father, a tall fair-haired man, sweat running down his face, who has just stumbled into the A & E department holding her.

'She has asthma,' he says in a foreign accent. 'It's got very bad.'

I lead them straight into the resuscitation room and over to a trolley. As the father tries to lay her down on it she refuses to let go of him.

'Papa,' she says tearfully.

'It's OK,' I say, gently disentangling her arms from his neck. 'What's your name?'

Nicki, the nurse, tousles the girl's fair hair. 'Dad's right here,' she says, pulling the father round to stand on the far side of the trolley so we can get on with things.

'She's called Solveig,' says the father, trembling and putting his hand on his daughter's shoulder. He stares intently at her face and mumbles something to her that we can't understand.

She is a thin, pale seven- or eight-year-old with blonde hair cut in a bob and a sharp nose. Her chest is expanded and rising in and out so rapidly that she reminds me of a bird.

Panic is contagious.

With shaking hands I attach an oxygen probe to her finger. She snatches it off, afraid, I think, that it will hurt. I put it back on and restrain her from removing it until she realizes it's painless. She submits. The probe shines two light frequencies through her finger; the amount that emerges on the other side will tell us the percentage of her red blood cells that are loaded with oxygen. I pull the back of the trolley forward so she's sitting up. I pull out and attach a child's mask to the piping, switch the oxygen on to the maximum flow and put the mask over her nose and mouth. Just before I put the oxygen mask on her face the finger probe produces a blue number on the monitor: Solveig's oxygen levels are 88%, confirming what we can tell from her shallow breathing – she is in real danger.

'Can you get the salbutamol and ipratropium?' I say to Nicki, who is already at the medicine cupboard.

With the oxygen mask on the blue number blips up and up until it settles at a relieving 97%.

'You'll be safe with us, Solveig.' Something I only say when I'm worried.

The consultant's tied up with another patient and Joe, the registrar, the most senior doctor around, has bustled in aware of the fuss. He asks the father what happened.

'We're . . . we're . . . we're on holiday here from Sweden.'

His pupils are flared with adrenaline, his forehead raked with fear.

'Her asthma's been bad for the last few days. Today we've been giving her lots of the . . . you know . . . the . . . the . . .' He tries to get his panic under control.

'The Salbutamol?' Joe asks.

'Yes, Salbutamol,' the father says.

I'm listening to Solveig's lungs through a stethoscope while the conversation is taking place, hearing their voices amplified in my ears. I try to fade the men out and concentrate on the sounds in Solveig's lungs. There is a worrying lack of air flowing with each breath, and plenty of the musical crackling and wheezing that tells me her small airways are inflamed and closing down to block the passage of air.

'But her asthma just got really bad, really quickly,' I can hear her father saying in a muffled faraway voice, through the quiet popping and whistling in Solveig's lungs. I unplug the stethoscope from my ears and now her father's voice becomes clear and close.

'We were in an aquarium right round the corner and they told me the hospital was just over the road so I just ran here.'

Nicki already has a plastic chamber that she has been filling with two liquids. She attaches it between the tubing and the mask on Solveig's face and the oxygen begins to blow the medicated steam into Solveig's lungs. The steam will relax the tubes in her lungs and help her to breathe.

'She wants to be a marine biologist,' her father says, following some internal train of thought. Then I notice he is looking at the paintings on the wall of the children's resuscitation room cubicle that depict the portholes in a submarine, through which can be seen colourful fish with bubbles emerging from their mouths.

'I got her a fish tank for her birthday next week; she's going to be eight . . .' He tails off. He looks drained, the adrenaline subsiding.

He has brought his daughter to us; now we need to save her.

Solveig pushes the mask away. I hold her hands to stop her

from pulling the mask off. It's easy to stop her, not only because she is young but because she is tiring. A bad sign.

The nebulizer gives off its calming, rasping hum, wafting its medicated steam into Solveig's lungs and I feel my heart rate subsiding. I look at the shallow rise and fall of her chest and just hope her lungs are shipping in enough gas to get the medicine where it's needed.

'Let's get some steroids,' I say to Nicki, who is already doing it, dropping the tiny pills into a small quantity of water.

'Has she ever been in hospital before with her asthma?' Joe the registrar asks.

'Several times when she was younger,' the father replies.

'Has she ever ended up in intensive care?' he asks.

'Once when she was small. But she's seven now and in the last few years things have been pretty good.'

'What tends to trigger the asthma?' Joe asks.

'Oh . . .' Her father frowns, and deep grooves rake his forehead again as he tries to get his tumbling thoughts under control. 'Dogs . . . colds . . . a lot of things. I don't know whether it's the pollution here . . .'

There's not much to do while we're waiting for the medication to do its job. Joe is asking the father about Solveig's medical history: other medical problems, medications, allergies, family history. Her father mentions that she has a twin brother with hay fever but otherwise there are no more details in the medical history.

I look at Solveig's pale intelligent face. I can imagine her nose pressed against the glass of an aquarium, absorbing the colours and movements and life stories of the exotic fish. I imagine her climbing trees with her brother, racing with him, being competitive. Then I look from Solveig to the blue number on the monitor denoting the percentage of her blood that is saturated with oxygen. In horror I see it begin to drop from 96 to 95 then to 94.

I look back at Solveig to see how she's doing. Her eyes are closing, her breathing is very shallow indeed. I put the stethoscope back on her chest. There is even less air flowing in and out than before we started the nebulizer.

'It's worse,' I say.

Joe grabs the stethoscope to listen and frowns. I take the muscle running from Solveig's neck to her shoulder and pinch it hard, she moans and opens her eyes.

Joe looks deep in thought. This shouldn't be happening; the medicine should start helping straight away. And despite the high fraction of oxygen we're giving Solveig through the mask the blue number on the monitor is still dropping: 93, 92, 90, 89. She is simply not getting enough gas into her lungs for the oxygen to reach her bloodstream in big enough quantities. If the levels keep dropping, her heart will stop due to lack of oxygen and she will die in front of us.

After five seconds' thought Joe reaches one arm out to a red 'pull button' on the wall behind the bed and tugs it outwards. Immediately the red button lights up and an alarm sounds at an urgent pace. Dee-dah-dee-dah-dee-dah.

I flick a glance at Solveig's father's face and wish I hadn't. The colour has entirely drained from his skin. Not a muscle twitches; he looks frozen to the spot.

I look at Joe, who is taking a pulse from Solveig's wrist. He looks as if he is struggling to collect his thoughts. *Damn*, I think. He's the most senior person here.

Dee-dah-dee-dah-dee-dah, the alarm keeps ringing. I try to do some thinking myself. The nebulizer is still rasping away, puffing out its magic steam. But the sound no longer calms me down. And the steam seems to be seeping into the room, and not into Solveig's lungs where it's needed.

Joe must be thinking along the same lines. 'Let's switch to a bag-valve mask,' he says.

Nicki grabs a clear-plastic lozenge-shaped balloon and attaches it to the oxygen. Galvanized, we swap over masks and I start squeezing on the balloon. Now we can try to force the highly oxygenated air into the child's closed-down lungs rather than rely on her breathing it in.

I squeeze slowly and firmly. There is a lot of resistance but some of the gas is getting in. I feel calmer now I have something to do, so I try to think. What did the dad say about her asthma not normally deteriorating this quickly? Is the asthma a coincidence? Has something else happened as well? I try to think of other things that rapidly compromise people's breathing. Is there a blood clot in the lung? Has she swallowed a foreign body, a coin or something?

The number on the monitor shows 93, then 92, then 90.

Dee-dah-dee-dah-dee-dah, sounds the alarm.

'Shall we get an X-ray?' I ask the registrar, who is also staring at the numbers. He winces as if my query rams home the fact that we may not have time for an X-ray before the young child in front of us dies.

We need treatment. But treatment for what?

'Could she have swallowed something?' I ask the father.

'What?' he says almost abstractly. He suddenly looks very old. His face slack and expressionless. He is here physically but mentally he seems a million miles away.

'Could she have swallowed something?' I say. 'A sweet, or a coin, or something.'

'A coin?' he asks, staring at his daughter who is ghostly white and scarcely breathing.

'Anything?' I say. 'Could she have swallowed something?' But I'm losing confidence in this whole foreign-body theory, after all I could hear quiet crackly air in both lungs as you'd expect in asthma; wouldn't a foreign body result in a different, more rasping sound or no sound at all? And Solveig's father is frozen to the spot, seemingly not computing what I've asked him.

Despite me squeezing hard on the balloon, the number on the monitor is now down to 84, then 82.

Solveig's eyes are closing. *Where the hell's the help?* I think.

Then people begin to arrive, other junior people at first. One of them helps Nicki attach heart-monitor pads. We have a pulse, too fast, but we have one. Then the anaesthetist wanders in, trained to be calm in situations when everyone else is losing their head.

She eyes up the monitor. 'What's the story?' she asks.

'Asthma,' Joe responds. 'Tiring, quiet chest.'

'Do we need to intubate?' the anaesthetist asks.

She reaches in a drawer and pulls out the kit she would need to place a tube down Solveig's throat. Then she takes the plastic balloon from my hand and starts squeezing. 'Quite a lot of resistance,' she says.

Even through the practised calm of decades of experience there's a strained tone in her voice impossible to miss, just the faint echoes of a thought that some people – even in well-equipped hospitals in the richest countries in the world, even children who want to be marine biologists with their whole lives ahead of them – some people don't make it.

'We need to intubate; we need a line and we need some intravenous salbutamol,' she says.

She has taken over. It's a huge relief.

Joe remains at the foot of the bed, nominally running the show but defeated. Another doctor grabs a cannula.

Nicki walks round to the father at the other side of the trolley, puts her arm round him and says, 'Do you want to stay while we do this or would you like to sit down over here?'

He is rigid, gripping the edge of the trolley in his hands. He seems organically attached to the equipment, like a tree growing out of the side of a ravine.

'She was eating a sandwich,' he says eventually.

'What?' I ask.

'You asked me if she'd swallowed anything . . . She was eating a sandwich.'

'A sandwich,' Joe mumbles.

'Did her breathing get worse before or after the sandwich?' I ask.

He looks at us, confused, desperately trying to remember. 'After,' he says finally.

Joe and I look at each other and a possible explanation for what we have been seeing, a possible key to the uncrackable code of her breathing, hits us at the same time: anaphylaxis. There's no rash, no swelling, but sometimes there isn't.

Now we can finally read the dying girl we have a solution.

'Nicki, we need an IM injection of one in one thousand

adrenaline, nought point three mils,' Joe says, suddenly invigorated.

Nicki goes straight to the anaphylaxis kit. She pulls out a small glass syringe and hands it to me.

'We need to give her an injection, Dad,' I say.

Nicki pulls down Solveig's trousers to expose her legs. I stick the needle in and press the adrenaline into her thigh muscle. She is so sleepy that she doesn't flinch at the needle. Neither does her father, who is stuck in his position gripping the edge of the trolley.

The anaesthetist looks at us quizzically as she is squeezing the plastic balloon. The blue number on the monitor is stuck at 78–79%, but at least it's not dropping.

A hollow needle is pushed into Solveig's hand and a line attached. Through the line we push in an antihistamine medication and then a steroid, all intended to work to reverse an allergic reaction. Then we drip in fluid.

We're doing something, and Joe and I now think we're doing something that will work. But how long will it take? Maybe we're wrong and this is a terminal asthma case.

'So her asthma was bad but it suddenly got worse after the sandwich?' I ask again to reassure myself.

'I guess so,' says her father. 'Yes.'

And at that moment it looks as if some colour comes back into Solveig's cheeks. She coughs a bit. The anaesthetist squeezes on the bag, purses her lips and nods in a positive way. We look at the monitor; the saturation figure starts rising: 81, 82, 84.

I can't restrain breaking into a grin. I look over at Joe, a small smile flickers on his face.

Solveig's father is still stuck there to the side of the trolley, looming over his daughter.

I put my hand on his shoulder. 'She's getting more oxygen into her lungs,' I say.

He remains still and then suddenly releases a huge exhalation, two vast lungfuls of air.

Solveig coughs again, opens her eyes and looks at us all and the strange scene she finds herself in, terrified. Then she sees her father and reaches for him. 'Papa,' she says.

He breaks his grip on the trolley, bends down to kiss her on the cheek and murmurs some words into her ear that we don't understand.

Diplomat

Adriana sits and stares sullenly down at her big leather boots as her mum starts in on all the things that are going wrong with her.

'She's disrespecting me all the time, ignores everything I ask her to do, slamming doors, saying – excuse me, doctor – the F-word to my face. She's disrespecting her aunt, who's like a second mother to her. She's fighting with her older sister and older cousins; she's physically fighting with them . . .'

At this Adriana smirks to herself.

Veronica is standing up, bouncing back and forth on her feet as she talks. Behind her is a noticeboard covered with posters about everything that can go wrong in life and the contact details of people who might be able to help.

'You see how disrespectful she is,' Veronica continues. 'The school are worried about her. She's stopped doing her homework. She speaks back in class. She's been in detention three times this term already. The school are wondering if she has ADHD, doctor. And she was never like this before. She was the perfect student. I really thought she'd be the one from the family to . . . to make it. She's fourteen and it's a bad time to be failing at school.' She pauses for breath. 'Then – I don't care; I'm going to say it to the doctor, Adriana – she's round her boyfriend's house the whole time, morning noon and night –'

Adriana interrupts the flow and shoots her mother a look

of disdain. 'He's a boy and he's my friend,' she says in a voice with a disdainful drawl. 'He's not my boyfriend. That's not the same thing.'

She has black trousers and a school jumper on. She's holding a yellow woollen hat in her lap and large red headphones clamp her neck, from which the faint sound of a synthesized voice and jangly guitars emerge. Above her head hangs a copy of a portrait of an eighteenth-century Spanish diplomat. Up on a shelf to the side are small plastic models of a brain, a spine and a cervix that I sometimes use for illustration purposes with patients.

'You see, doctor? You see the lip I get when all I want is to help her.'

'Adriana, can you turn the music off?' I say, and she reaches slowly into her pocket and presses something and the headphones fall silent.

Veronica seems satisfied that Adriana has responded to my request. She looks at me, raising her eyebrows. 'She's fourteen years old and I don't know what they get up to,' she says. 'I don't know what's going on, and –' here she takes a big intake of breath – 'since her father went back to Brazil I don't know how to control her.'

Adriana is grimly staring at her boots and rolling her eyes.

Veronica flings her arms out dramatically. 'Doctor, I'm worried about where this is going to end,' she says, more to Adriana than to me.

I'm just trying to work out in my head where to start when Adriana speaks up sarcastically.

'Have you finished?' she asks her mum.

Veronica looks at her. 'For the moment, Adriana, for the moment.'

'Well, will you leave so I can talk to the doctor alone?'

Her mum flinches as if she has been physically struck. Tears spring to her eyes and she quickly looks away from Adriana as if to obscure this. The make-up on her handsome face cannot obscure the worry lines on her forehead and the dark circles around her eyes.

Even sitting down it's clear that Adriana is already taller than her mother, gangly and loose-limbed. And she seems the calmer of the two, sitting there while her mother can't keep still.

'You see, doctor, what I have to deal with?'

I frown neutrally.

'But I think perhaps that's a good idea,' I say to Veronica. 'Then Adriana can talk to me openly.'

Veronica looks frightened, as though I have picked a side.

'And afterwards we can all talk together,' I add.

'If you could talk some sense into her,' her mum says pleadingly, picking up her red-leather handbag from the floor, 'and try to work out what's going on with her.'

As Adriana watches her mum leave the room, her face doesn't show any mercy. As soon as the door closes she turns to me and looks at me cautiously, as if to say, now what am I going to get from you?

'It sounds as if things are difficult,' I say.

'Uh-huh,' she says.

'Tell me,' I say, acting as if I have all the time in the world.

We sit in silence. Up until this moment Adriana has seemed tougher and more streetwise than her mother. Now she suddenly looks like a child.

'I'm depressed,' she suddenly says in a quiet voice, all trace of attitude vanished. She sits very still.

'Tell me about it,' I say.

'I've been depressed for three years.'

'I'm sorry to hear that.'

'I can literally remember the day it started.'

'What happened?'

She shakes her head. 'Nothing. I'd spent the weekend at my aunt's house with all the women in my family and my mum had picked me up and we were driving back through the town and I suddenly felt this . . .' She is twisting the yellow hat in her hands. 'It's hard to describe,' she says, looking up at me to check I'm following.

'It was like a pain in the stomach, as if nothing would ever be the same again. And it's been here ever since.'

We sit in silence while she collects her thoughts.

'It's been getting worse,' she continues. 'Last Christmas we went back to Brazil to see my dad. Me and my dad were swimming out in the bay when I felt the current was pulling me out.'

She stops speaking again and swallows hard. Tears are brimming on her lower eyelids and she is looking straight ahead of her as if to keep them balancing there as long as possible.

'When I realized what was going on I began swimming out to sea.'

I give an understanding nod, even though the only times the tide has pulled me out I've been frantic to get back in. She looks incredibly vulnerable in her adult body. 'You wanted to die?' I ask.

She fiercely wipes at her eyes with her sleeve. 'I think so.'

We sit in silence again.

'What happened?'

'My dad swam out and dragged me back in.'

'How did you feel when you got back to shore?' I ask.

'I was totally exhausted. I didn't get out of bed for a few days. I told my parents what had happened and they arranged for me to see a psychiatrist.'

Why didn't your mother mention this? I wonder.

'Was that useful?' I ask instead.

'A bit. He asked me lots of questions and then he told me that this is a difficult time of life for everyone.'

She looks at me challengingly. 'I felt a bit better for a few days, but then I felt empty again. Then, later in the holiday, I put on my dad's clothes.' She looks at me keenly, to clock my reaction.

'Right,' I say, nodding, not really sure where this is going. 'OK. What happened then?'

'I felt calm. I felt happy for the first time in years.'

'I see,' I say. 'And since then?'

'That's how I feel every time I wear male clothes. Happy,' she says.

Adriana explains to me that she stole some of her dad's clothes and since they got back from their trip she has been routinely putting them on in the privacy of her room, and this same feeling of peace always steals over her.

'What do you make of this?' I ask.

'I don't know,' she says, smiling for the first time. 'I've been looking all that trans stuff up on the internet, but I don't know . . . What do you think?'

What do I think? I look up at the portrait of the diplomat above Adriana's head. It's a beautiful oil painting, copied by a transgender patient of mine from an eighteenth-century original. The diplomat looks intelligently and calmly out at the world from a soft fleshy physique that has been painted then faithfully repainted. He is resplendent in fine blue, gold and white garments with a hint of red trim, a book held in one hand. His expression is hard to read. His mouth is smiling but his eyes are not.

We have a number of transgender patients at the surgery, and, as is the way with medicine, we see more of the cases where it hasn't gone well. The painter of this portrait is still on a difficult journey.

'Can I ask you some more questions before I answer?' I ask.

Adriana raises her eyebrows and half smiles at my evasiveness.

I laugh along, then I ask her about her family. It seems they all came over from Brazil when Adriana was a toddler. All she can remember from her few years there is a smiling grandmother, now dead, and her grandmother's pet parrot, who is still alive. Adriana's parents would argue a lot; her father was a musician and money was always tight. She felt closer to her father and she felt her mother became jealous of their relationship. Her parents are nominally still together, but for the last five years her father has been living and working in Brazil, which means Adriana only sees him twice a year.

Adriana feels anger at her father for leaving, even though she kind of understands his reasons for doing so. 'He couldn't get work here, and I think my mother drove him crazy.'

Now she is in a house with her mother, older sister and brother, aunt and two female cousins. Adriana feels pity for her mother and her aunt, who is divorced.

'They're obsessed with men, but they've been treated so badly by them. It's kind of pathetic. I hate listening to them talk about it.'

And when her mother is vitriolic about her father, as she often is, Adriana gets enraged and argues back on his behalf.

At school Adriana finds it difficult to engage with the other girls who she generally finds superficial, obsessed with appearance and emotionally highly strung. She hates the dynamic between the sexes at school, in particular the sense of boys and girls judging her on how she looks. She generally dislikes the pressure she feels to dress in a feminine way and leans as masculine as the uniform rules allow.

She's been getting periods for a year and doesn't like the way she feels emotional when they're coming or the way they mark her as female.

She has a male friend, Robbie, who she can tell everything to, and she likes to spend time with him.

'He's open-minded and he lets me try on his clothes.'

'And do you get the same sense of relief from putting on his clothes?'

'Yes,' she says.

'What does Robbie think?' I ask.

'He thinks we should all be whatever we want to be,' she says.

'And what do you think about that?' I ask.

'I don't know.' She screws up her eyes. 'I mean, perhaps he's right . . . I dunno.'

'Is he your boyfriend?' I ask.

'No.' She shrugs. 'I don't really care much about that sort of thing.'

We sit in silence for a while.

'What do you think your mum would think if you told her about this?' I ask.

'I've told her,' Adriana says.

I'm surprised. In her spiel earlier Veronica mentioned a lot of things, but neglected this one.

'What does she think?'

'She thinks it's like a fashion thing,' Adriana says, rolling her eyes in mock despair. 'She doesn't get it.'

'I imagine it's a challenging thing for a parent to hear,' I say.

'I guess so,' Adriana says.

'I think your mum wants the best for you.'

'I guess so,' Adriana says even more quietly than before.

'Everything she said earlier, her level of concern, told me she cares deeply about you,' I say.

Adriana looks at her boots and nods, then looks up at me. 'So what do you think?' she says.

I look up at the diplomat on the wall. 'I don't have the answer,' I say.

She looks at me carefully.

'But you've told me you've been depressed for three years, and that you might have tried to kill yourself, and I take all of that very seriously. I think gender is a very complicated thing,' I continue. 'It has a physical side, a psychological side and a cultural side. And all of this is supposed to be agreed upon in one body.'

Adriana looks down at her leather boots and smiles. Perhaps because I have failed to give her an answer.

'What were you hoping would happen next?' I ask.

'I guess I'd like to talk to somebody about all of this,' she says.

'I think that's a good idea,' I say. 'We should start with the general mental health team, look at it all. Shall we get your mum back in and make a plan?'

'Yes,' says Adriana.

Adriana's mum is hanging around the waiting room,

talking frantically to somebody on her mobile phone. She immediately rings off as she spots me waving and comes back to the room. This time she accepts the seat I offer next to Adriana, right under the diplomat. She looks questioningly at her daughter.

'Thanks for being so patient, Veronica,' I say, and quickly summarize everything that Adriana has told me. When I mention the relief Adriana feels when she dresses in men's clothes a look of alarm crosses Veronica's face.

'What do you think about this?' I ask.

Adriana has an ironic smile on her face as if armoured up for the onslaught. But Veronica sits there silently for a while, and when she speaks she is calmer.

'I think it has a lot to do with how things are between me and her dad.' She sighs. 'Unfortunately Adriana's been around a lot of arguments in her life.'

She turns to her daughter. 'I'm sorry for that, Adriana,' she says.

Tears spring to Adriana's eyes and she aggressively wipes them away.

'Sure, I understand,' Veronica says blankly. 'Who wants to be a woman in this world?'

She suddenly seems very young herself.

'But being a teenager is a very confusing time. And, Adriana, when you get an idea in your head you can be very stubborn. You know that. You get that from me. And I'm just frightened of what might happen if you get stuck on this idea. I'm just frightened that things might happen that are permanent and everybody regrets.'

When Veronica says this Adriana looks frozen to the spot and a look of fear crosses her face. 'We're a long way from thinking about anything permanent,' I say. 'I think we should start with a referral to the general mental health team to assess Adriana's mood along with everything else.'

Veronica sits and thinks about it for a while. 'That sounds OK, doctor,' she says.

'I told Adriana that it's obvious to me how much you care for her,' I say.

They stand up, Adriana looming over her mother. Veronica puts a hand on her shoulder but Adriana shrugs her off.

The long-dead diplomat stares out of the portrait with penetrating eyes, a faint smile on his face.

Veronica picks up her bag and walks out of the room. Adriana follows, careful to walk a little to one side.

Happiness

'Who's gonna win the Cup Final?' the boy asks.

He is a youthful fourteen-year-old – looks more like twelve – with a thatch of mousy hair. He looks right on the cusp: at the end of childhood and at the foot of the ladder to manhood.

'I dunno, Gareth,' I say honestly. 'Who is going to win?'

'Man City!' he says, a grin lighting up his face.

I can't help but smile back at his naked enthusiasm. 'Do you, by any chance, support Manchester City?' I ask.

'Yesss,' he almost shouts.

Gareth has a bit of a lisp because his tongue is somewhat big for his small mouth. He has a pointed chin and a short neck. His upper eyelids drop precipitously across the sides of his brown eyes by his wide flattish nose, like slightly drawn curtains.

'We're a long way from Manchester, Gareth; can I ask why you support them?'

'Because they're the best,' he shouts, and he weakly punches an arm up into the air with enthusiasm. The effort of this seems to exhaust him, and he puffs and pants a bit and settles back into the pillows.

His mother looks on with concern from the sofa that doubles as a bed for parents staying in the children's hospital. She and I are wearing plastic aprons, and I am wearing latex gloves in an attempt to reduce the number of germs Gareth comes into contact with.

The bedside cupboard in which Gareth's Manchester City dressing gown and slippers are stowed is bristling with get-well cards, most of them football-themed. Nets bulge with goals, players wheel around with shiny white grins, rows of spectators reach for the heavens.

'You must be one of their biggest fans,' I say.

Gareth smiles again but he's knackered. 'Yesss,' he says quietly.

'Well, I look forward to celebrating with you when they win,' I say.

'Do you support Man City?' Gareth asks.

'Definitely,' I say, 'at least for the next few weeks.'

This seems to satisfy him.

'What else do you like, apart from football?' I ask.

'I love chicken,' he says, his smile widening further.

'I like chicken too,' I say. 'Fried chicken with chips especially.'

Gareth looks confused.

His mum laughs from the sofa bed and puts down the work papers she has been reading and annotating. 'Gareth, explain to the doctor who Chicken is.'

'Chicken is my dog.'

'Oh,' I say, laughing. 'You lucky thing, having a dog.'

'We called her Chicken because she used to be scared of everything,' his mum says.

'I cured her,' Gareth says.

'How did you do that?'

'I talked about it to her,' Gareth says.

'Well done,' I say.

'She's very cuddly,' Gareth says. 'She's my special friend.'

'Nothing better,' I say.

'I can't cuddle her now,' Gareth says. He yawns deeply. He looks exhausted. 'I'm not allowed to.'

'Just while you're on this treatment, Gareth,' his mother says from the sofa. 'After that you'll be able to cuddle her as much as you like. She's a very licky dog,' she explains to me.

'The best kind,' I say.

'Gareth, do you mind if I talk to the doctor?' his mother asks.

Gareth is dropping off to sleep in the bed and he smiles as his eyelids flicker and droop.

Gareth's mum Fiona is wearing a grey business suit. She puts down her work papers as she stands up. 'Could we go outside to talk?'

One of Gareth's parents is with him all the time. They take it in turns. That and looking after their two other children and both working high-powered jobs, shuttling back and forth from their home, which is thirty miles away.

We walk out of the side room into the tiny vestibule that acts as a kind of germlock to the ward outside. We can see through the glass window into Gareth's room that his eyes are closed now and that he hasn't noticed us leave.

I stand with my back to the sink. We are a few metres apart, with Gareth through the window on one side and the bustling ward through the door on the other. A strain comes across Fiona's face as she prepares to speak. She's had too many chats with too many doctors bearing bad news and she has to steel herself at the prospect of exposing herself to more.

'I wondered if you could tell me how we're doing with the chemo?' she says.

'Well, I think it's early,' I say, 'and I'm not the ideal person to talk to, but at handover we were told he's doing fine.'

I look at her; she looks as if she wants to hear more.

'I guess at this early stage it's all about how he's tolerating it. Later we'll find out if it's been effective.'

'I want you to be honest with me.' She fixes me with grey eyes. 'Gareth has been very unlucky in his life, with the Down's syndrome, and heart problems when he was a baby, and then the leukaemia, and the other chemos not working. He relies on me and his father to protect him; we need to know everything.'

She looks at me penetratingly with her gaze. 'Everything,' she repeats. 'We know this is our last chance, so please don't try to spare me.'

'I won't,' I say. 'Genuinely. We heard he was doing fine with it. We'll be checking bloods twice a day to make sure the destroyed tumour cells aren't poisoning his bloodstream. But so far so good.'

'And why did I hear a nurse talking about antibiotics this morning?' she says, trying to keep a waver from her voice.

I'm taken aback. I don't know anything about that. I fish the crumpled handover list from my back pocket, find Gareth's name on it and read the cursory notes.

'I think she was probably referring to the spray we're using to try to prevent him getting an infection of the mouth. There was no mention of active infection this morning.'

I look at her to see if she is reassured by this junior doctor reading out from a printed list.

The deep furrows in her brow relax a little.

'Shall I ask Doctor Rossi to come and talk to you later?' I say.

'Yes please,' she says. 'I know she's busy, but whenever she can. It'll be my husband after three o'clock so she can talk to either of us.'

I scribble a note on my list. We both look through the glass window at Gareth. He's sleeping soundly, dwarfed by the mound of pillows, snoring away. He is so innocent that it's hard not to smile just looking at him.

'I think it's amazing how hard you both work to be with him,' I say.

'It's exhausting,' she says. Her face is pale and drawn. 'It is exhausting. We didn't find out he was Down's until he was born,' she says. 'We owe him so much.'

We stand there for a while but she doesn't elaborate. After a minute, I leave to go on to the next patient.

Later that afternoon I stop by Gareth's room. Gareth is awake, and seems to have more energy. He's playing a top trumps card game about deep-sea creatures with his father, David.

David is slim, with a salt-and-pepper beard and wire specs. He is holding a Japanese spider crab between his forefinger and thumb. 'I challenge you on size,' he says to Gareth.

'Size, Dad?' says Gareth, beaming from ear to ear. 'Are you sure?'

'Yes, size,' says David. 'Is there something wrong with that?'

'Size,' says Gareth again, chuckling. 'No, nothing wrong.'

David lays the Japanese spider crab on the bedcover. It sits there, monstrous legs and feeding arms splayed out.

'Four metres,' David says, holding his arms as far apart as they can go. 'This crab would fill this room, Gareth; what do you say to that?'

'I've got bigger,' he says.

His dad laughs. 'Bigger? Bigger than this gigantic crab?'

'Yes. I've got the card you're scared of.' And he lays down a great white shark on the bedcover. 'Six metres, Dad, six metres.'

He looks at his dad, a huge smile creasing his face.

'Not the great white,' says David, trembling with fear. 'Oh no.'

'I win,' says Gareth in triumph.

'But the great white, that's just cruel,' says David. 'I should never have watched that film,' he says to me.

'Don't worry, Dad,' Gareth says and he strokes his father's arm. 'They don't come on land, Dad; you'll be OK with me.'

There's a knocking at the vestibule window and we can see Dr Rossi waving hello. She pokes her head through the door. 'David, could I rescue you from the great white for a moment?'

A look of genuine fear flashes across David's face.

Gareth has noticed. 'Are you OK, Dad?' he asks, grabbing his father's hand.

David squeezes Gareth's hand and smiles. 'I'm fine, love.'

Gareth relaxes. 'Don't worry, you might win the next one.'

'I don't know, Gareth,' says Dr Rossi, 'I'm not sure anyone can beat you at this game.'

Gareth beams with delight.

While David goes out to talk to Dr Rossi I play a few hands of deep-sea trumps with Gareth. Gareth knows the cards backwards though he can't pronounce all the names. His coelacanth – a large primitive-looking fish – is bigger than my sea pig – a translucent pink many-legged helium-balloon-like creature that stalks the ocean floors. His dumbo octopus – so called as it looks like a flying elephant – is freakier than my acorn worm, a phosphorescent swimming phallus. His giant oarfish, a sort of sea serpent, swims deeper than my twelve-metre-long basking shark.

'What do you think it sounds like down there?' Gareth asks.

'Deep in the ocean?'

'Yes.'

'Pretty silent, I reckon. Some whistles and squeaks from the whales. What do you think?'

'Dark and cold. I wouldn't like to go there,' he says, and shudders. 'Would you?'

'Mmmm, not without a friend,' I say.

Out in the vestibule Dr Rossi has been reassuring David that the chemo is going fine, so when he comes back in he has a spring in his step.

'Gareth,' he says, 'stop beating the doctors; you might need their help one day.'

It must be a month later when the crash call goes off at three in the morning and I find the bleep telling me to go to the cancer ward and am horrified to see a hive of activity focused around Gareth's room. I've been working with different teams in the interim and through the vestibule window, as I'm whipping on the plastic gown and gloves, I can see how different Gareth looks now. He is gaunt and his skin has a blueish tinge. His eyes are closed but I am relieved to see that he is moving his limbs and breathing. On the sofa bed next to him his dad, David, is sitting up. He's wearing tracksuit bottoms and a T-shirt, looking shell-shocked.

'His blood pressure is very low,' the nurse says, quoting

me figures. 'He's already on tazocin and itraconazole for chest sepsis.'

'Hi, Gareth,' I say. 'How are you doing?'

He's feverish and weak and mumbles something with half-closed eyes.

We set up some fluids and drip them gently into his circulation. The intensive care doctor arrives, a slight Indian lady. She asks us what is going on and has a look at the notes. She sits down with Gareth's dad on the sofa that he was just sleeping on.

'Has there been a discussion about whether it's in Gareth's best interests to go to intensive care?' she asks.

'We've talked about it with Doctor Rossi before,' David says, 'and we've always wanted everything possible to be done for him but . . .' He pauses and looks at his son, now unconscious again in the bed. His voice becomes husky. 'We do know that there could come a point when it's not the right thing to do.'

The intensive care doctor is listening to him intently.

'OK. And currently, if I understand correctly, he's on the last possible chemotherapy. All the other ones have failed.'

'Yes,' his father says. Uttering the word seems to cause him physical pain.

We recheck Gareth's blood pressure and it seems to be improving slightly with the fluids, his skin becoming pink again. It's decided that he's stable enough to stay on the general ward.

We bleep the cardiologists to come and scan Gareth's heart. Infections can cause low blood pressure by many means, but we also know that this chemotherapy can affect the function of the heart and that Gareth has had heart problems since birth. If his heart is failing, along with the chemo and the infection this could well be too much for him.

We call Dr Rossi who always wants to know when her patients are unwell and she sets off to come into the hospital. Gareth's father phones his wife and asks her to come in as well. With Gareth asleep and stable for the time being I offer to make him a cup of tea.

He follows me into the canteen for patients and parents. It's been decked out to look as little like a hospital room as possible with a check tablecloth and framed cartoon prints of animals, TV stars and football players on the walls.

'It's the Cup Final tomorrow,' he says. 'Gareth is very keen to see it.'

'I remember,' I say, pouring boiling water on to the tea-bags. 'He's a big Man City fan.'

A strained smile crosses his father's face. Everything wonderful about Gareth must feel painful; he's been on the edge of the abyss for so long, and now he's at risk of disappearing inside.

'Have you got children?' he asks.

I nod and tell him briefly about them.

'Gareth was our third,' he says. 'We were really struggling as a family before he came along; there were some things, some problems between me and Fiona.'

I offer him milk and he nods, then accepts the cup.

'And Gareth, with all the problems he had and the way he took . . . the way he takes all of it in his stride, with nothing but gratitude, he . . .'

He stops with his mouth open as if not sure what to say next, rubs his brow, then takes a swig of tea.

'He showed us that almost nothing we thought was important was important,' he says, and has another swig of tea.

We fall to talking about other things, unimportant things to give him a break from his agony.

When we get back to the room again the cardiologist is there, a large man looming over Gareth with his echo machine. He runs the rubberized half-moon probe over Gareth's bare chest, slick with contact gel, and on the screen you can see hazy images of the chambers of his heart, lazily contracting and expanding. The cardiologist presses some buttons and now the blood within the chambers lights up on the screen as either red or blue depending on whether it is travelling away or towards the probe. Another few buttons and he can get a measurement of the blood flowing out of the left ventricle, the final chamber of the heart. At my enquiring glance he just shakes his head. He checks a few more things, then carefully wipes the gel off Gareth's chest and the probe and takes the machine out of the room. The nurse rebuttons Gareth's pyjama top and tucks him in.

When Gareth's mum arrives Dr Rossi heads off to the family room with both parents. A while later they troop back into his room. We can see that all of them, including Dr Rossi, have been crying. His mum and dad go over to the bed and sit next to Gareth, one on each side like outriders, stroking his head while he sleeps.

They take him home later that morning, to his sisters, his grandparents and his dog Chicken. It's arranged so that nurses will meet him there and set up medications to keep him comfortable.

Later that afternoon at home I wake up haunted by bad dreams. I turn on the TV to see young blue-shirted football players running around the pitch, leaping over advertising hoardings in the prime of physical condition, huge grins all over their faces. Small huddles of players in red stand hugging each other in consolation, tears streaming down their faces.

I've missed the Cup Final.

Manchester City won three–nil.

Youth

Aztec Priest

Later the police break down the door to Pete's room and find unsent letters expressing the anguish and bewilderment that he had been carrying hidden from the rest of the world. Later his family say they had no idea he was suffering, and we are left pondering the capacity for humans to hide their pain, like hermit crabs sheltering most of their entirety inside a borrowed shell.

According to friends and family he had been acting normally – a happy-go-lucky seventeen-year-old with a winning smile, a good son, a painter, a lover of animals – right up until that night when the horrible passion suddenly spilled out.

None of this preamble is known when Pete arrives at the hospital with his kingly retinue, on a trolley flanked by paramedics. Deep self-inflicted stab wounds weep red on to his T-shirt. Pulseless throughout his time on the ambulance, despite CPR and adrenaline shots. Face pulled back in a rictus grin.

The savagery has a galvanizing effect. He is conveyed to the resuscitation room and has clothes sheared off, lines drilled into his shin bones and blood poured in, oxygen thrust down his throat, ribcage cut open and flipped back in a clam shell, his aorta clamped and his heart gripped in the hand of the on-call surgeon – like an Aztec priest propitiating the gods – and rhythmically squeezed in an effort to get blood to circulate and buy time to start exploring and fixing the wounds.

Because he is young he is worked on for a long time. The full resources of the state at his disposal. And throughout that hour he, the patient, remains still and silent, offering no response to the brutal stimulation. The only one of us unconcerned by this ritual of regret. He is dead throughout, and he remains dead until it's clear that he will not be reclaimed, and time is called, and looking around I see numbed and exhausted faces.

Pete's friends arrive at about that time and are to be seen running in jagged lines through the emergency department, tearing at their clothes and weeping, unable to contain the frenzy inside.

Female. 18. Back Pain.

In a Herculean feat the night team have emptied the entire
A & E. The eerie quiet of the department and the morning
winter light filtering through the high tinted windows make
it resemble a fish tank.

I sit alone in a glass-walled booth, staring meditatively at
the computer screen with its unnatural expanse of flickering
whiteness. Then a patient silently drops on to the screen.

Female. 18. Back Pain.

I walk round the corner.

In the middle of the cubicle a young woman is standing
up, shifting her weight from foot to foot. She is scarcely an
adult. Her skin is smooth and she's wearing a baggy denim
men's shirt, her hair pulled back in a black bun. Her pale face
is clear of make-up and taut with pain.

It's sad for someone so young to be afflicted by a problem
like back pain, I think sentimentally. She looks the picture of
health, but she can't keep still because of the pain, and there
is a look of fear in her clear blue eyes that surprises me. She
looks trapped. Unable to escape the pain. Perhaps she's losing faith in the body she used to trust.

'Do you want to lie down, Rachel?' I ask.

'No thanks,' she says, a grimace in her quiet voice. She has
stopped moving around now.

'More comfortable standing?'

She nods.

A young man with a scraggly beard and braids in his long hair is sitting on the bed, a woven bracelet on one wrist. He has a look of deep concern on his face. I ascertain that he is her boyfriend.

'How can I help?' I ask brightly.

'My back really hurts,' Rachel says, and she looks ashamed and scared.

'She's in a lot of pain,' her boyfriend says testily, and Rachel shoots him a look as if to tell him to shut up.

'When did this pain start?' I ask.

'Saturday,' she says.

It's only Wednesday now, I think. *Four days. Why come to A & E? Why not go to the GP?*

'And did you fall or damage your back before the pain started?'

'No.' She shakes her head. 'I was at work on Friday, but I didn't hurt my back.'

'What work do you do?' I ask.

'Behind a bar.'

'And you didn't strain your back in some way, carrying something?'

'No,' she says. 'They had me pulling pints all day.'

'Have you taken any painkillers?'

'Yes,' she says.

'Are they helping?'

'Not really,' she says.

'We've been to the doctor's about this twice already,' says the boyfriend in an aggrieved tone. 'We went to the minor injuries unit on Saturday night and they just gave her paracetamol, then we went to the walk-in health centre on Monday and they gave us codeine. It hasn't helped.'

He looks strangely defeated by this as if he didn't expect life to throw him a girlfriend with four days of insurmountable back pain into his path so soon.

Jesus! I think. Back pain, and this is their third visit to seek medical attention in five days; no wonder the health service is on its knees. Why should I be able to sort out this problem any more than the previous two people, and how long will they wait before they go to seek a fourth opinion?

'Did the codeine help at all?' I ask Rachel, a cajoling tone in my voice, hoping she'll say yes, as I'm fully aware that I have little else to offer.

'Not much,' she says. 'It's actually getting worse.'

And again I see that surprising fear in her eyes.

'And we're supposed to be going travelling to South America in a few weeks,' the boyfriend says.

'Have you had back problems in the past?' I ask Rachel.

'Yes,' she says with something that looks like relief. 'I fell out of a tree when I was younger and I had some problems with it then.'

'Does it feel like it used to?' I ask.

'No,' she says, looking concerned again, 'it's different.'

'Can you point to where it hurts?' I ask her.

She gestures behind her.

'Can you show me exactly by pressing on the spot?' I say.

She hesitates for a long time and I feel the institutional impatience of the emergency department coursing through me.

'Is that OK?' I ask, unclear why she is being so slow.

Reluctantly Rachel unbuttons the denim shirt and turns away to show me where the pain is. For half a second I see her body in profile as she turns and I can see that her belly is protruding like an oversized rugby ball. Then she has turned fully and is facing directly away from me.

'The pain is here,' she says, bringing both hands up behind her and pointing her thumbs into each side of her lower back.

'Right,' I say, feeling confused by what I've just seen.

'Are you pregnant?' I say to her back, wondering why no one has mentioned this yet, and feeling, for some reason, that I'm transgressing as I ask.

'No,' she says into the wall.

Now I'm completely taken aback.

'You're not pregnant?'

'No,' she says adamantly.

Baffled by this confirmation I look across at her boyfriend for assistance. He is staring at the floor. I cannot read his expression.

'OK,' I say, trying to collect my thoughts, 'so the pain?'

She points her thumbs into her back again.

'Can I press?' I say. She nods and I poke my fingers hard into the flesh of her loins.

'Does that hurt?' I say.

She shakes her head.

'OK,' I say. 'You can face me again.'

As she turns round I try to think things through, and again I'm flustered to see the unanticipated, unmentioned swollen abdomen.

'Look, you're sure you're not pregnant?' I find myself asking again. 'I mean, you look pregnant.'

'I'm not,' she says.

Her pale blue eyes flicker towards me, then away so she is staring up and out of the high window where the winter sun filters in.

My nerves are jangled by the whole situation. I feel a crushing weight of responsibility. Is she pregnant and suffering some awful medical complication? Am I being stupid and missing some classic abdominal condition that visually mimics pregnancy?

The emergency department is silent. I notice that Rachel has a silver teddy bear earring pinned to one ear. Her pale face is taut, thoughtful.

My mind grasps at straws. Perhaps the boyfriend, mild-mannered as he seems, is intimidating her in some way.

'Would you give us a moment?' I say to him.

He starts getting to his feet, as if more than happy to go.

'No, he can stay,' Rachel says hurriedly.

Then suddenly her face is convulsed with pain and she starts pacing up and down in the cubicle, then pausing and trying to get comfortable.

I look over at her boyfriend. I am struck by how young he looks.

'Has she been doing this much?' I ask.

'Yes,' he says.

'For how long?'

'For the last few days,' he says.

It takes about a minute for the pain to pass. For the entire time her boyfriend and I are silent and still, the low winter sun pouring in the window, the department silent as a church. Then Rachel stops pacing and rubs her swollen abdomen.

'When was your last period?' I ask.

She looks a bit confused. 'I don't . . . They've been a bit irregular,' she says.

'When was your last one?'

She mentions a month. I count forward to the present day. 'Nine months ago,' I say, raising my eyebrows, then turning to the boyfriend who has a look of defeat on his face. 'And how long has your belly been like that?'

'There's been a lot of bloating,' she says.

'How long?'

She shrugs. 'I don't know.'

'And have you felt any . . . any kicking in your belly in that time?' I ask.

She frowns. 'I'm . . . I'm not sure.'

For a moment I expect a TV crew to crash in through the curtain. I feel like I'm being tested as part of some psychological experiment. Her denial is so solid, so ridden with fear that I begin to get infected. Two medical professionals have seen her this week and treated her for musculoskeletal back pain. A significant part of me doesn't want to be humiliated by misdiagnosing pregnancy in a woman with back pain. But the belly?

'I think you're pregnant and in labour,' I say.

'I can't be,' she says.

'Why not?' I ask.

'I just can't.'

'What do you think,' I say to her boyfriend, 'could she be pregnant?'

He has his head in his hands. It's as if he is having a long hard think.

'I don't know what her mum is going to say,' he says finally. 'It's her birthday tomorrow; she's having a big party with caterers and a marquee.'

'I wouldn't worry about that,' I say.

'You don't understand,' he says, tension in his voice. 'Her mum went nuts when Rachel got her ear pierced.'

'I can't be pregnant,' Rachel reiterates. 'It's not possible.'

'Shall we do a pregnancy test to be sure?' I say, fixing her with my eyes. I need proof to break the thick glass of denial.

She nods but can't look me in the eye. I hand her a tiny clear plastic cylinder with an empty label on the side and she walks off to the toilets clutching it. They are the other side of the waiting room and as soon as they've walked off I begin to feel anxious about that 'no'.

I'm unsettled by the level of denial this couple are exhibiting. So deep it took in medical staff twice already this week. A denial foundering on the hard biological rocks of foetal development.

Suddenly I feel like I've done something dangerous in sending her off to the toilet on her own. Faint wisps of a lecture about concealed and denied pregnancies from medical school pass through my mind, all the scary stuff. The pregnant woman cannot accept the fact and so buries it into her subconscious. The depths of deception and self-delusion and the vulnerability of the unborn child are a frightening combination. I remember news stories I've read about foetuses being found in public toilets.

I look out into the waiting room towards where the toilets are. It's beginning to fill up with patients. The boyfriend is sitting on one of the screwed-down metal benches and I consider asking him to accompany her to the toilet. Then I tell myself to get a grip. The psychological precariousness of their situation has infected me.

Still I feel relief when Rachel comes back to the cubicle

with her boyfriend and says warily that she hasn't been able to produce any urine to be tested. She hands me back the empty plastic cylinder and for a second we are both holding it and at that moment I look directly into her pale, drawn face.

I think of what the average pregnancy contains: all the conversations, the books, the classes, the shopping, the tests and scans and appointments, the medical and family wisdom, the hopes and fears, the tears and laughter. All bypassed. Everything locked in this tense head.

'Rachel,' I say holding that cylinder, 'you've come to the right place; we'll look after you.'

No sooner have I said it than she walks a few steps and places her palms flat against the wall at head height underneath the high sunlit windows, sticks her rear out into the middle of the room and presses as if trying to push the wall of the hospital over.

'Let's get you to the maternity ward,' I say.

Her eyes are closed. 'Yes,' she says through clenched teeth, surrendering herself to the pain.

Her boyfriend gathers up his satchel and her cardigan for the journey and hovers at the edge of the cubicle. I want to give him a hug.

'And what happens next?' he asks.

At the end of the day I look up Rachel's medical record on the system. I'm surprised to see a discharge letter from the maternity unit has already been written with follow-ups arranged throughout the coming week with health visitors, a psychologist and social services.

Patient gave birth to a baby girl at 3.30 p.m.

Concealed/denied care. No antenatal services accessed. Arrived at A & E in labour.

Mother surprised but pleased to have a child. Grandmother available to help with newborn.

Reviewed by psychologist on ward. They are happy to discharge.

We wish her all the best with her daughter.

The Outsider

'Tariq,' I shout over the hubbub of the waiting room and a thin, intense-looking young man stands up.

It's the Sunday evening of a scorching bank holiday weekend, and the waiting room in the emergency department feels like a sauna. It is teeming with the summer day's casualties: sunburnt, drunk, drugged and battered people slumped across the rows of chairs. Several hold T-shirts to head wounds. Everyone is shiny with sweat. I can feel liquid rolling down my spine to the small of my back.

Suddenly there is a jarring peal of trumpets, which organizes itself into the mariachi opening strains of 'Ring of Fire', which is terminated as a man answers his phone. 'Five hours, mate, not a word of a lie . . . Nah, it's jokes, mate, jokes.'

As Tariq threads his way with dignity through the crowded waiting room, kempt in trainers, jeans and a drenched linen shirt, he looks extremely solitary. He has waited for hours in the packed roasting waiting room to see a doctor, despite being told by the triage nurse that because he is not suicidal he is wasting his and our time.

He shakes my hand politely, apologizes for the sweat on his palm, and thanks me for seeing him as I usher him into the main department and a small bare cubicle.

When Tariq sits down he stares carefully at the floor and jiggles his right foot up and down. He explains that he has been feeling anxious and depressed for years, but his anxiety has become worse in recent months and weeks. The standard A & E position on low mood and anxiety is that if you're not feeling suicidal you should go away and see your GP with whom you can develop a useful therapeutic relationship. The department is so rammed that I am tempted to simply reiterate this advice, but Tariq has waited and so I decide to hear why.

'It's a different level now,' he says. 'I can't focus on anything, can't even read a book. I've lost touch with all my friends because I find it hard to be around them.' He stares intently at the floor. 'It takes me hours to get to sleep, and a few hours later I wake and spend the rest of the night worrying.'

'Anything happened recently to make things worse?' I ask.

Tariq looks up at me for the first time, sweat dripping down his face, eyes bulging. 'The world,' he says. 'Isn't the world just a terrible place?'

'What do you mean?'

He looks at me as if about to say something risqué. 'Look at what's happening in Iraq, Kashmir, the Democratic Republic of Congo. Men, women and children being killed and maimed. The rape, the torture. It's . . . it's unbearable. I can't get the images out of my head. The bombs dropped from overhead. The ISIS videos . . . have you seen them?'

'No,' I say, and feel sweat running down my spine.

'They decapitate people,' Tariq tells me. 'They burned a man to death in a cage; they drowned a guy in a fish tank. This is what I'm talking about. This is what the human race is?'

'Maybe you shouldn't watch those videos,' I say. I'm shaken by his fervour, his animation, and the truth of what he's saying.

'You're right . . . you are right . . . but I can't stop myself because I know it's happening whether I watch it or not. And it's not just that. It's knowing that it's going on at this very moment everywhere. Landmines exploding into a million fragments and ripping off the legs of children, and –' here he stares up at me accusingly – 'someone placed that landmine, someone sold it to that person, someone manufactured and marketed it.'

'Yes,' I say. 'That's an awful thought.'

'And here,' he continues, 'here in the street the way people treat each other, the way they look at each other, barge past each other, everyone's trampling over everyone else to get ahead. I'm really struggling to cope with it.'

My eye is caught by a poster with cartoon pictures of doctors, nurses and porters promising zero tolerance to patients who ASSAULT, ABUSE OR HARASS HOSPITAL STAFF. The humans in the cartoons have vivid hairstyles but completely blank and featureless faces.

'And it's so damn hot,' Tariq says, tugging at the shoulder of his drenched shirt, 'through our greed and stupidity we're making the planet burn. Why would anyone want to live in a world like this?'

'Are you feeling suicidal?'

He shakes his head. 'I wouldn't kill myself. I'm too scared for that.'

I ask him all the usual questions about low mood and anxiety, delusions, hallucinations, obsessions. The answers I get are unenlightening. I ask him about work and establish that Tariq has quit his job manning the grill of a kebab restaurant. Now he gets by on some dwindling savings.

'Any mental health problems in the family?' I ask.

Tariq looks at me sharply as if I am some sort of mind reader.

'Yes,' he says carefully. 'My dad suffered from depression.'

'Suffered?' I ask, narrowing my eyes.

Something runs across Tariq's face. He sits in silence for a moment, thinking.

'He killed himself when I was a young kid,' he says finally.

We let that sit there for a while. Through the blank blue cubicle curtain we can hear the hum and buzz of the department, the bleeps of machines, the shouts of a drunk.

'I'm very sorry to hear that,' I say. 'Do you remember him?'

'I think so,' he says, his face twisting with pain. 'I remember him bouncing me on his knee. I've seen photos of him since. My mum tells me he'd been depressed for years, then they split up . . . He hanged himself. He was the same age I am now when he did it.'

Tariq is deep in his thoughts. 'I've been thinking about him a lot recently,' he says. 'Can't stop. Whenever I see a man in the street of a similar build I find myself looking at their faces to see if it might be him. And I have dreams, where my dad is talking to me in a house, telling me something important. Then we walk outside and there's no gravity so we float up into the air and I realize that there's nothing to stop us from rising up out through the atmosphere and off into space.

'Am I going mad?' he asks.

I ask a few other questions to which the answers are 'no'.

'You don't seem psychotic,' I say. 'I just think you're under a lot of stress at the moment. People are often haunted with thoughts of mortality when they reach the same age at which a parent died. Are you in touch with other family members?'

'My mum moved back to Pakistan,' Tariq says. 'I see her once a year. My brother moved to the States years ago; we've fallen out of touch since he found Islam.'

'Are you religious?'

He pulls a face. 'Are you?'

'No,' I say. 'Brought up that way, interested, but not a believer.'

We sit in silence again. This is A & E; I'm never going to see this man again. What can I do but sympathize and suggest he sees his regular doctor?

'What were you hoping we could do for you today?' I ask.

He looks at me, sweaty face, goggling eyes.

'I needed to ask someone . . . to ask you. How can you get up in the morning with all of this going on?'

I pause. The question is outside of the textbooks, which is a relief in some ways, as I'm new to the A & E job and sick of being asked medical questions I can't answer. But having no right or wrong answer it's harder to know what to say, so I say what I think.

'First of all,' I say, 'it is hard to disagree. The world is an appalling place, and if you pack together a small fraction of the daily horror it's hard not to drop into a depression. There have been times when I've thought much the way you do, just wanted to pull the covers over my head. The Germans have a word for it, *Weltschmerz*, world-pain.'

Tariq looks at me. Now he's really listening, really concentrating. Is this why he sat in that godawful waiting room for six hours?

'What I'm trying to say, is that you're not alone. Lots of us feel or have felt like this.'

'But how can you cope with it?'

'Well,' I say, 'there are wonderful things in the world too. And I guess I've chosen to focus on those.'

'What things?' Tariq asks.

'Music, laughter, nature, love, friendship, sex, children.'

'Do you have children?' Tariq asks.

'I do,' I say.

'And you were happy to bring them into this world?'

'I thought a lot about it,' I say.

He chews on this evasive answer for a while.

'I hope you don't mind me asking,' he says, 'but isn't it unbearable that all of that is going to come to an end with death?'

Now it's my turn to pause, to fade out the mayhem through the curtain and focus.

'It can feel that way,' I say, 'but I figure it makes no sense to be upset about that future when we have the thing in front of us right now.'

'I guess you must see a lot of misery here,' Tariq says. 'Doesn't that get you down?'

'The opposite, actually, within the misery we see people's drive to live, to get whole, to enjoy life again.'

Tariq reflects on this and seems satisfied. 'Thank you,' he says. 'Thank you very much, doctor.'

I smile. 'I don't think I've done anything. And I'm not saying these things are easy or expecting you to feel the same. So what I suggest you do is get to your GP as soon as possible and try to arrange some counselling. We need to get you back in some sort of ease with the world. Perhaps a short course of an anti-anxiety medication as well. Of course I'll write to them about what we've talked about here today.'

For no real reason other than to have something to jot on the hospital form I feel Tariq's pulse and am surprised to find that it's a bit fast. Listening to his heart with the stethoscope I can hear it clattering away behind his ribs. So I take

his blood pressure and it's higher than it should be in someone of Tariq's age. Probably the heat and stress, I
rationalize.

'Any caffeine, nicotine, or recreational drugs today?' I ask.

'No,' he says, 'I never take any of those things.'

'I know it's a stupid question given what we've been talking about,' I say, 'but are you feeling anxious now?'

'Much less so now we've spoken,' he says, 'but I guess I'm
always anxious.'

'Well, that's probably why your pulse is fast,' I say, almost
to myself, mulling it over, and it is damn hot in here. I can
feel the sweat running down my chest. But a thought has
dropped into my head.

'Look, as you're here and you've waited so long, why don't
we do a blood test just to check you're not anaemic and that
your thyroid gland's not misfiring. They'll probably be normal, but then at least we know.'

'OK, why not?' Tariq says, almost as if to please me.

I take the blood sample and explain that it'll be an hour
before the results come back.

'I'll wait outside,' he says, 'but I want to thank you. You've
helped so much. Honestly I feel so much better after talking
to you. Just to know that I'm not the only one who has felt
this way.'

I get carried away in the whirlwind of the shift seeing sunburnt, alcohol-drenched, beaten-up patients, and it's an hour
and a half before I check the blood results. To my surprise
they are not normal. Tariq has an excess of thyroxine in his
blood. This raises the metabolism, and can cause sweating,
weight loss, a fast heart rate and, perhaps most pertinently,

anxiety. The thyroxine helps our internal fires burn, and Tariq's are being stoked higher and ever higher. I have been assuming Tariq's negative thoughts, his tragic history, his *Weltschmerz*, have been colluding to affect his physical state, when conversely a glitch in his physical fabric has probably been driving his psychological state, putting him in perpetual fight-or-flight mode. And there's another conundrum in the test results, as they seem to suggest the reason for this excess thyroid hormone lies not in the thyroid gland itself but in the pituitary gland in the brain. The most common cause of that in someone his age is a brain tumour.

I steel myself to deliver this troubling news to Tariq's already anxious brain and walk back to the teeming waiting room and call his name again. Lots of red-faced people turn and look at me then turn away disappointed. But no Tariq. I scan the room but can't see him. I repeat his name louder. A short man gets up and tries to pretend that he is Tariq as a way of being seen quicker but I tell him to sit back down.

I walk outside the hospital where the last of the summer-evening light filters through the vast plane trees. The night air is still hot and hordes of revellers are stumbling out of the local park and dancing in the road to a large boom box. I cannot see Tariq anywhere. I go back inside and call the mobile number we have for him on the triage sheet. *Damn, it's one digit too long.* I take off the last digit but the number doesn't function. For the rest of the shift I call Tariq's name in the waiting room and check the street outside before each new patient, but he never answers.

The next day is Monday and I call the GP surgery on Tariq's triage sheet, which is a long way from his home address.

They say he left them years ago and they haven't been asked to forward his info on to a new surgery. From their records they were not aware of any thyroid or pituitary problems. I play with the mobile number we have, dropping each of the digits in turn but on the few occasions I get a dialling tone the person on the other end does not recognize his name. I look online and find the phone number attached to the address Tariq gave us on the triage card. When I call it the person there denies ever knowing anyone of that name. As it's the only lead I have I write a cautious letter to the address – aware that someone else may open it – telling Tariq he must urgently register with his local GP and get them to repeat the blood tests we did because they show something significant. And then, sweating from the heat of the department, I move on to the next patient, and the next, and the next. On the way home from that shift and for the rest of that long hot summer I find myself looking for Tariq in the face of every tall man I pass, so I can tell him that he's carrying a tumour in his head that is stoking his internal fires to an unbearable temperature. Then autumn comes and I can no longer remember what Tariq looks like and his fading memory haunts only my dreams.

Transmission

I poke the hollow needle with its bevelled edge into the clapped-out young man's wrist where I felt his thready pulse a few moments before. To my pleasure bright crimson blood wells up through the needle in a bumpy rhythm and then with each beat of his heart a fine spray leaps out of the needle's open end and lands, sowing a field of poppies, on the white gauze carefully laid out below. That rhythmic geyser tells me I'm in the artery where I want to be, but the weakness of the spurt tells me his blood pressure really is low and I need to get on with it.

I pass a flexible wire, about the length of a pencil, back down through the needle into the artery inside. Now I thread the needle off and the man is left with a piece of wire sticking out of his emaciated wrist, marking the path into his radial artery. I struggle a little to pass a thin silicone sheath on to the guide wire. Sweat wells on my face; it's hot with the sterile blue gown, hat, mask and gloves on protecting the man from my germs. Eventually I do it, passing the silicone tube down the length of the wire and deep into the man's wrist where it will stay. Now it's the wire's turn to come out, and Tiago the nurse steps in to attach the monitor so we can get a second-by-second account of the patient's blood pressure.

As I move up to stand by the man's head, to place a line into his neck so we can drip noradrenaline into his bloodstream to give him a fighting chance of fifty more years roaming this planet, I see how deathly pale he is. His ribs are prominent beneath the thin cotton hospital gown, the small tufts of black hair on his chin and chest look pasted on, his arms and legs are stick thin and seem far too long for his small body. What has led him to be in this wretched state?

Down in A & E he was incoherent. Everything pointed to a raging infection. He had a high fever, a rumbling cough and when I pressed a thumb on his chest it left a bright white coin-sized imprint that took five seconds to regain colour, a sign that his circulation was failing. The rough-looking man who brought him in said he'd been unwell for over a week and refusing to go to the doctor. Instead he'd been at the man's flat smoking crack cocaine and crystal meth.

'He's called Nick,' the man said, smiling nervously to reveal brown teeth. 'I dunno anything else about him except he's got money. He seems posh, like. Oh, an' he's got a death wish.'

The man said he needed to go out for a cigarette and after that no one could find him. We reckoned fear of authority had got the better of him. Searching Nick's pockets turned up a few coins, cigarette papers and an empty plastic lighter. We had nothing to identify him with, but it was clear he was sick enough to need intensive care.

Now I'm standing at the head of the bed in the intensive care unit, city lights twinkling through the window behind my back, the needle hovering over Nick's jugular vein, when Tiago says, 'Look, doc,' and points at the red blood pressure trace on the monitor. The crimson waves are worryingly shallow, the beep-beep-beep familiar from so many hospital dramas is too fast.

I look down at Nick's gaunt face. The skull beneath the

skin. Lank strands of dark hair halo his bony brow. His eyes are closed; he has luxurious long dark lashes. For a minute I wonder if he's stopped breathing, but the oxygen mask is misting and the saturation levels are respectable given the thick consolidation we saw in one lung on his chest X-ray.

'Nick, Nick,' I say loudly into his ear.

He doesn't reply.

A jolt of adrenaline thuds through my body at his failure to respond. The hormone makes my heart beat faster and harder, my arteries contract, my blood pressure rise. The opposite of what I need; I'm jacked up enough as it is. *Fuck it!* It's Nick, whose blood vessels have become porous because of the bugs flowing around inside him – he's the one that needs the adrenaline. I feel my stomach constrict. I'm worried we've left it too late. And with Lin back down in A & E helping a sick child, and Ash on the other side of the intensive care unit dealing with an old man desperately trying to die it's up to Tiago and me to sort this out.

All this runs through my head as I'm poking the massive needle into Nick's jugular vein.

'Will you do a trap squeeze, Tiago?'

Tiago moves up to the other side of Nick's head and carefully reaches under the sterile drape on which my equipment sits and grips the muscle that runs across the back of Nick's shoulder and pinches it as tightly as he can.

Nick grimaces and mumbles something like 'gerrof'. Relieved by this sign that his brain is getting a certain flow of blood, I take a deep breath and continue my work. It's the same technique as at the wrist. Confident we're in the vein, because of the darker burgundy-coloured, less-oxygenated blood that fills my syringe, I do the threading and unthreading trick with wire and needle, but when I try to pass the thick silicone central line sheath over the top of the wire it won't go in, despite my shoving. Then I realize I've forgotten to open up the flesh and vein around the wire. I grab the scalpel and try to make a delicate slit around where the wire is protruding barbarically from Nick's neck.

I can sense Tiago tensing on the other side of the bed. I make the mistake of looking up at the monitor and can see Nick's blood pressure has dropped to a point where his heart could stop at any moment. Sweat drops into my eyes, obscuring my vision, and I wipe at my face with a gown-clad arm. I could ask Tiago to get a syringe of a drug to push through the cannula in Nick's hand to boost his blood pressure temporarily but drawing it up could take precious minutes. I curse the fact that we don't have it ready and waiting. Now what I need to do is just get this bloody line in. *He's only young, for Christ's sake.*

I grip the wire where it protrudes between thumb and forefinger and make one last nick with the scalpel. I feel an instant sharp flash of pain in my gloved index finger, then a welling up of wine-dark blood bubbling over Nick's neck – Nick's blood not my own. I shove the silicone sheath on to the wire with trembling fingers. This time it slides down into the core of his body to nestle by his heart. We do our last bits of fiddling and Tiago attaches the line with the precious noradrenaline and we start to push the drug into his bloodstream. We smile at each other, expressing relief after the panic we had been suppressing seconds before. But, hell, the risk, the adrenaline, that's partly why we're here at three in the morning in this high-tech eyrie high above the city.

When I finish by sewing the line into Nick's skin I'm

relieved to feel him squirming at the pain as the crescent-shaped needle bites into his flesh. I look up at the monitor and see the blood pressure rising, the red waves deeper. Nick has some more sea to swim in.

As I strip out of the gloves and gown I look through the window at the twinkling city lights below and wonder if one of them comes from the window of the bedsit where Nick was recently living. I inspect my gloved finger, the one where I felt the slice of pain and am surprised to see no evident tear in either the latex or in my skin.

At the beginning of the following night's shift we hand over in the glass office. This is surrounded by glassed-off bed bays, each containing a patient lying in a bed and a nurse sitting at a stool. The glass walls give off misleading reflections. They look like religious cells, with nuns and monks praying over the dying. The patients are almost all knocked out with lines delivering drugs, ventilators delivering oxygen, and monitors that tell us their vital signs in primary colours, monitors that we have to remind ourselves not to look at in place of the patient. It's as if the monitors contain the patient's soul while the body waits in purgatory.

When the day registrar gets down the list of patients to Nick he says, 'So this one's not doing so great. Still requiring fluids and norad, still acidotic. His oxygen sats keep wavering but we've managed to avoid tubing him so far. We still just have a first name so no medical history, but we do know he has AIDS.'

There is a murmur of surprise at this last comment. 'I know,' the reg continues, 'not a word you hear much these days. Luckily someone thought the chest X-ray looked dodgy and did an HIV test and he's positive and clearly untreated. His CD4 count is ridiculously low and viral load sky high. We've started antiretrovirals and antifungals, so hopefully he'll start doing better.'

I remember the slicing pain when I had my fingers in Nick's jugular vein and stare intently at my index finger, but I can't see a cut. And there was no cut in the glove so I'm safe. Aren't I? I force myself to concentrate through the rest of the handover but it's a bit of a blur until I get a grip and manage to push the thought of my finger to the back of my mind.

When I come to Nick on the ward round his skeletal form and wispy beard remind me of those marble sculptures of Jesus Christ taken off the cross. Lines and heart-monitor pads where the stigmata should be. Tiago tells me he's scarcely communicating, just the occasional grunt or groan. I listen to his chest and it's still horribly congested. The lines on the monitor tell me that with most of advanced medicine's technology deployed on the battlefield we are still struggling against an army of bacteria, fungi and viruses to free the immune system they have taken hostage.

When at four in the morning the crash call bell goes off I get a sinking feeling as I recognize Nick's room number 23 flashing up on the screens. When I get to the bedside Tiago is squeezing on a large green rubber balloon attached to the mask over Nick's mouth, forcing the oxygen-rich gas into his lungs. The patient is no longer strong enough or intact enough to breathe for himself.

'His sats were dropping,' Tiago says.

When I take over I can feel the resistance of Nick's lungs when I squeeze. They are tight and rubbery with all the fluid and pus generated by the infection. Ash arrives and prepares the gear to put Nick into a deep artificial sleep. Tiago clicks a button and the vast window that gives on to the ward immediately becomes opaque. It's as if we're doing something shameful.

As I squeeze the pearly white propofol into the line Ash is up at his head with the tube. He perfunctorily speaks into Nick's ear, 'We're going to put you to sleep for a while.'

Nick is pretty far gone and this is the only sensible medical course of action. Still it feels enormous sending someone to sleep knowing it could well be a one-way trip, pulling the plug on their last moment of consciousness.

Tiago has readied the ventilator and everything goes smoothly. Another machine takes over another bodily function.

After Ash goes off and I'm writing up a drug on the chart Tiago speaks.

'You know, Tom, before he went off he seemed to perk up a bit. He opened his eyes; I thought we were going to have a conversation. I know this is crazy but it looked as if he stopped breathing on purpose.'

I shrug, thinking perhaps the stress is getting to Tiago. 'Well, we're in control now. He doesn't have any choice.'

Tiago presses a button to unfrost the glass observation window. I look at Nick's chest, rigidly rising and falling under the ventilator's command and I remember what the man who brought him in said: 'He's got a death wish.'

Now we're in charge, I think. *What else can go wrong?*

Nothing until the next night.

At handover we still have no background information on

Nick. It's a big city, easy for someone who wants to disappear into a bedsit to smoke drugs to do so effectively. The day registrar tells us that Nick is requiring less noradrenaline to keep his blood pressure stable. Often a sign that someone's turned a corner. It's the fourth of four night shifts for me and I always feel jumpy on the last one, a little overexcited at the prospect of escape.

On ward round my time is taken up by a sick liver-transplant patient who requires regular transfusions of platelets to stop him from bleeding to death and a delirious middle-aged man recovering from having half his bowel removed trying to jump out of bed and pull all his lines out. So it's a bit of a sucker punch when the crash bell goes off at five thirty and I see room number 23 flash up on the screen.

I get there to see Tiago flapping around and the blue line on the monitor tells me why. Although we have taken over Nick's breathing with a ventilator his oxygen levels are plummeting rapidly into the death zone. We probably only have a few minutes to sort this out before cardiac arrest. But what is going on? For a moment I am mesmerized by the monitor, where Nick's fate looks as if it is playing out.

'One moment his sats were fine, and then they weren't,' says Tiago.

His panicked voice snaps me out of my fugue. I try to get my fatigue- and adrenaline-addled brain to take a rational approach. The ventilator is chugging away, attached to the central hospital oxygen supply and registering good oxygen levels and high pressures as the gas passes through. The breathing tube is attached to the ventilator and looks to be in precisely the right place at the patient's lips, so up to this point everything seems to be operating normally. Then we look at Nick, and despite this high-pressure gas seeming to pass deep into his throat his chest is not rising and falling as it should. I grab a stethoscope to listen to what is happening in Nick's lungs. Not very much of anything is going in and out. Not a situation conducive to life.

'Let's take over,' I say, detaching the ventilator from Nick's breathing tube and attaching the green floppy balloon instead. Tiago runs the oxygen tube through this and I squeeze the balloon. Damn, it's hard to get anything into the lungs; there is massive resistance somewhere in the breathing tube or somewhere below in the major airways of the lungs. But to happen so rapidly? Squeezing hard we get the chest to rise a bit and the oxygen levels begin to come up a touch.

Ash turns up, also summoned by the crash bell, and I explain what is going on.

He has a squeeze of the bag. 'We have to reintubate,' he says.

This time there's less faff as Nick is knocked out already. Ash makes it look easy. The breathing tube comes out and a new one goes in.

'That's going in much better,' says Tiago, after reattaching the balloon and squeezing it.

'The old tube was in the right place,' says Ash, tying the new breathing tube carefully on Nick's mouth. The blue oxygen levels on the monitor rise back up to where they should be.

I hold the old breathing tube up to the light and squint through it. There's a huge plug of orange mucus blocking it with only a hole of a few millimetres through the middle.

The mucus must have been pulled from his inflamed lungs into the tube plugging off the airway.

'We were asphyxiating him,' I say.

I'm back thirty-six hours later for the weekend day shift. The night team hands over to us in the glass room. There's a congenial atmosphere with a larger team and autumn sunlight streaming in the windows. The consultant has put some Miles Davis on, to help us think, he says, and brought in a box of doughnuts for coffee time. We're told that Nick's condition has stabilized and he's ready to come off the ventilator. 'His sister's here,' says the night reg. 'Can someone talk to her and find out what they can?'

I make my way to one of the family rooms. There's a large print on the wall, which was donated by a family member in gratitude for a patient looked after here many years ago. It depicts a farmer ploughing a field on a cliff, oblivious to Icarus plunging into the sea below. Underneath it, sitting on a low sofa, is a woman with ginger hair twisted into dreadlocks and a freckled face. She's skinny and pale and wearing a jade-green dress that matches her eyes.

Her name is Lisa. She explains that she got a message via a social media account yesterday saying her brother was in this hospital. It seems word got out through some of his drug-taking mates and eventually reached someone who used to be at secondary school with Nick and Lisa and who sent the message to her.

Lisa shows me a picture on her phone that shows her sitting in a bar with a man who loosely resembles Nick. It's shocking to see him filled out, tanned, healthy. In the photo Nick has his arm round another younger man, with tight curly hair. There is pride in Nick's grin and a wild look in his eyes that have reflected red in the camera's flash.

'How is he?' she asks.

In loose terms I describe how unwell he's been. Lisa sits looking at me, her mouth taut, refusing to betray emotion. When I tell her Nick seems to be pulling through, a single tear wells up and drops unhindered down a freckled cheek.

'We used to be very close,' she says, looking at the picture on her phone. 'I haven't seen him for a few years.'

I shrug, as if to say it happens. 'Do you have any other siblings?'

She shakes her head. 'It's just me and him.'

'Any other family?'

'Parents.'

'Do they know that he's here?'

'Neither of us are in touch with them.' She turns her piercing green gaze on me. 'Do you know anything about what's been going on with him?'

'Until now we only had a first name,' I say, 'and he hasn't been in a position to talk. It would be useful to know some of his history.'

She takes a deep breath and goes back early. 'We had a difficult childhood. Our parents . . .' She tails off. 'We had to learn to stand on our own two feet from a young age. I tried to protect him but . . . he was chubby, shy . . . When he realized he was gay he swore me to secrecy. He didn't trust them. They were old-fashioned.'

She pauses. 'I was worried about him when I went off travelling. But I wanted to get away as well. It was so horrible at home. Nick told me to go. "Blaze a trail for me," he said. When I came home to visit he had transformed. He'd come out. Our parents were horrified. He'd lost weight. He'd become very striking. He was a real . . . queen. I was so proud of him . . . I spent a lot of time in India. He always said he'd come out and join me, but he never did. I realize now our lives went on to separate tracks when I left him behind . . .

'He moved here . . .' She waves her hand to take in the sprawling city below. 'At first we'd meet up whenever I came back and he was doing OK; he was high on his new life, but he was partying a lot and in an intense way like he was trying to exorcise his demons. Then he got in with a dodgy crowd. Too many drugs, not enough sense. At some point he got infected with HIV. After that Nick stopped wanting to meet up. I said I'd come back to help him but he said he was fine; the treatment was keeping him well.'

'How long ago was this?' I asked.

'Oh, seven, eight years ago. A year or so later I hooked up with him in a bar. He seemed . . . he seemed happy for the first time. Not exhilarated any more, but happy. He had a boyfriend called Leon. That's him,' she says, pointing at the other man in the picture. 'Younger than him. Didn't take drugs. And Nick was sweet with him. I could see for the first time he'd found someone to protect. When I went off to India that year I felt happy about him.

'About nine months later I heard that they'd split up. Nick didn't tell me why. A year later we met and he was drunk and high. He told me he'd infected Leon because he hadn't been taking his meds and he'd lied about it. Apparently Leon was sick with the HIV, and not responding well to the medication. That happens, doesn't it?'

'Sometimes,' I say. 'It's very unlucky.'

'From then on it was full self-destruct mode for Nick,' she

says. 'He started hitting the drugs hard. So hard he wasn't taking the meds properly. I tried to be sympathetic, to help, when I was back. Tried to get him to come out to India with me, to dry out. He couldn't look me in the eyes. Eventually he stopped answering, and I stopped trying.'

I can smell the guilt. Nick's, hers.

We sit in silence for a while staring out over the city. Helicopters buzz through the greying skies, sirens distantly howling. I think about what the man who brought him in said about Nick having 'a death wish'. And about what Tiago had said about him stopping breathing on purpose. Surely fanciful.

Now that Nick is awake the real healing has to start.

'Would you like to see him?' I say at last.

She stands to follow me.

'I should tell you he's been through a lot,' I say. 'He looks pretty terrible. And he may be confused when he wakes up. He's had a lot of medications washing through him.'

When we get to the bedside Nick is breathing by himself, no tube in sight, and he's propped up on pillows, eyes half closed. The red, blue, green and yellow lines on the monitor say that everything is fine with him. The illusion of control.

I go to the side of his bed. 'Hi, Nick. I'm one of the doctors who's been looking after you.'

He nods, eyelids still low.

'Your sister is here to visit,' I say. 'Are you well enough to see her?'

He opens his eyes wide. They're a piercing grey colour, and he looks up to take in his surroundings and the ginger-haired woman hovering at the foot of the bed. 'Lisa,' he says in a croaky voice.

She cautiously walks round the side of the bed, avoiding the line emerging from his skinny wrist.

'Hi, Nick,' she says. 'How are you doing?'

He grabs her hand tightly. 'I wanted to die,' he says, tears welling up in his eyes. He holds on to her hand with his bony fingers.

She stands there for a while crying openly. Then she whispers something in his ear that sounds like, 'Don't leave me behind.'

The Bent Knife

When the emergency department red phone goes off for the sixth time that day the evening shift is on its way into work and the day shift is tired. The message the ambulance crew delivers over the phone is simple: a stabbing, patient conscious, distressed, vital signs normal. We ready ourselves as best we can by calling an anaesthetist, warning the surgeons they may be called upon to operate, and arranging the equipment we might need. The A & E consultant, a cheery Geordie, tells us that we've managed plenty of stabbings before and that whatever happens this will surely be our last patient.

Twenty minutes later the trolley is wheeled in through sliding doors by two paramedics, letting in a blast of wind and several orange-coloured leaves that swirl and whirl before settling on the shiny white lino floor. Lying on the trolley is a slim young white man with brown curly hair wrapped in a silver marathon runner's blanket for warmth, collar and blocks splinting his neck, a hugely swollen right eye. Trailing in his wake are two policemen in stab vests.

The trolley is wheeled next to a gurney in one of the resuscitation bays and the patient is slid across on a sheet. Probes are attached to the man for heart trace, pulse, breathing rate, blood oxygenation and pressure. The patient is quiet and still apart from the occasional gesticulation with his right arm.

Our consultant winks at the shorter and older paramedic. 'What have you got for us today, Derek?' he asks.

Derek cocks his head on one side. 'Probably a stabbing. Found him lying on his back. Conscious. Head like this. Vital signs all stable on the journey but he's not moving his left side much. He was in a lot of pain so we gave him ten migs of morphine. The police were there first.'

The taller policeman takes up the story. 'A postie saw him staggering around by the canal and then collapsing but didn't see anyone else around. By the time we got there he was lying on the towpath. He seemed to be in a lot of pain. There was a small patch of blood on the floor. The knife was next to him. We don't know if he's been stabbed with it, or if it's his and he was punched or hit his head when he fell.'

'This is the knife,' says the short red-haired policeman. He holds up a clear plastic bag with what looks like a large steak knife. It has a wooden handle and a six-inch blade with one straight edge and one gently curved serrated edge. Two other details are striking. The blade is coated in dried blood to the hilt and one inch of its tip is bent sideways as if it has met with considerable resistance at some force.

'Anyone else been reported stabbed?' asks the consultant sharply.

'Nothing's been radioed in,' says the tall policeman. 'No perpetrator has been found; no other stabbing's been reported.'

'Then we have to assume it's this lad.'

The A & E consultant asks the man how he is. He answers with a moan of pain and a sweep of his right arm.

The red-haired policeman makes to speak, checks himself then decides to speak anyway. 'He was talking when we found him. He kept saying this one word, "Sun, sun, sunny", over and over again.'

'Any idea what that meant?' asks the A & E registrar.

'We asked him but he just kept repeating it.'

The patient's left arm doesn't move. His right eyelid is massively swollen and blood gently seeps around it, staining the right side of his head a purplish colour. The doctors try to ignore the eye: it looks like a painful wound, but it's not going to kill him. Instead the A & E consultant initiates a call and response to assess how critical his state is and how first to act.

'Airway?'

'Clear,' says the anaesthetist.

'Breathing?'

'No compromise,' says the registrar after listening to the man's lungs with his stethoscope and checking his oxygen levels.

'Circulation?'

'Pulse and blood pressure stable,' I say, looking at the monitor.

This category incorporates the heart and blood vessels. Presuming that the knife with the bent tip was used on him we need to locate the stab wound. A nurse cleans away the blood from his head. No underlying wounds are visible, just this tightly swollen region encompassing the right eye with seeping blood. His sweater, T-shirt, jeans and underpants are quickly snipped off with a pair of shears and the front of his naked body is scrutinized, then, after a coordinated *log roll*, his back. No wounds are seen, and no obvious fractures to explain the lack of movement in the left side of his body.

I insert a plastic tube into a vein in his right hand and

draw off blood to be sent for testing. While I'm doing that the rest of the team has moved back to the checklist.

'Disability,' barks the consultant, meaning he wants us to focus on the patient's nervous system. Now we're back to the eye. The registrar tries to open the swollen lids. The man moans in pain. The eye shows white underneath, the pupil contracting at the sudden ingress of light. Everything is so bruised and swollen it is hard to be sure if there is a stab wound here or not.

The morphine seems to be wearing off. The man is groaning and thrashing his right arm in distress. The decision is quickly made to sedate and intubate him and get a CT scan of his head.

The anaesthetist draws up a drug to make the man's muscles go slack and another to stop the conscious part of his brain from working. Once these have been pushed into the man's veins and he is limp and asleep, his throat is forced open with a blunt metal hook and a flexible plastic tube is fed down his windpipe, secured and attached to a portable artificial ventilator the size of a small rucksack. This is placed on the bed between the patient's legs.

The man is wheeled on a gurney into CT Room 2 followed by doctors, nurses and the red-haired policeman clutching the plastic bag with the knife. The patient is transferred across on to the narrow bed that forms part of the CT scanner. He is strapped down on to this narrow-mattressed gutter, the head end of which sits at the middle of a massive perpendicular doughnut-shaped machine. The rest of us pile through a door into the small CT scan booth, a large radiation-proof window looking back into the room with the patient in the scanner. A radiographer taps at her computer.

This commands the scanner to slowly slide the patient on his mattress so his head enters the doughnut, which then takes a series of X-ray pictures from three different angles to help answer the fundamental question of 'What is wrong with this person?' Sitting between the patient's legs the portable ventilator mechanically inflates and deflates his lungs.

While these machines do their work we have a moment to rest. The consultant starts talking about the violent machete injuries he saw when he worked in South Africa. This seems to be in part an attempt to discourage speculation about what has happened to the patient, but it's hard not to dwell on it. Was it a drug deal gone wrong? A fight that got out of hand? An attempted execution? A random attack? Could the patient have in any way anticipated that his Wednesday would turn out this way?

The consultant has moved on to talk about the different bullet wounds he has seen. He is just explaining that the poorer quality the gun, the more higgledy-piggledy a bullet exits the barrel and the worse damage it tends to do, when suddenly he's cut off by the radiographer saying, 'Here it is.'

Now there's silence in the booth. Inside CT Room 2 the ventilator mechanically sucks and blows to keep the man alive. Meanwhile everyone in the booth cranes for a look at the computerized representation of his head on the computer screen.

The CT-scan images are presented in three different planes. You can scroll through pictures of the head transversely – as if you had finely sliced the patient from the crown to the neck and were looking at the inside of the slices – seeing first the top of the head and then a two-dimensional image of every 5 mm of the skull and brain down to the neck. You can scroll through the pictures sagitally – as if chopping the patient's head lengthways – starting with the left ear and moving into the head (along the ear canal) towards the midline (where the nose is) and then out of the right side of the head, ending with the right ear.

But in this case the only visible wound is the right eye so our radiographer goes straight for the coronal images – as if you were looking straight into the man's face and using a peeler to pull off slices of the man's head from front to back.

The radiographer manipulates the images so we start with the tip of the man's nose, then drop 5 mm further into his head with each image. The front of his face, the eyelids, the air cavities behind the nose, and, lower down, the jaw and teeth, then a few shots that take in the eye globes themselves, which look to be mercifully intact. But there is a two-centimetre-wide black line that shouldn't be there. It starts above the right eye globe, like an internal eyebrow, and we see that it persists as we scroll deeper into the man's brain, heading back and slightly upwards towards the midline and penetrating the grey and white matter until it terminates at the inside of the top of the skull. We sneak glances at the knife in the plastic bag and the bend in the thick metal blade tip.

The CT scan tells us that he has been stabbed above the eye, through the brain, with such violence that the knife appears to have bent on the inside of his skull. None of the brain structures that keep us breathing and the heart beating are in this area, but the bits that make us who we are – our movements, our sensation, our control, our personality – all these are in the firing line. But scans will not tell us what the effect will be on him; we will just have to wait and see when he wakes up.

There is silence in the booth. I wonder at the mentality of

whoever did this, of the person who plunged a knife into a man's brain with such force. What turn of events led to this knife tip being bent on this skull? In the next room the ventilator draws and blows.

'Well, there it is,' says the consultant finally. 'Man's inhumanity to man.'

The neurosurgeons are called to review the images. They need to make a decision on where the patient should go: intensive care or the operating theatre. The patient's vital signs are checked again. While we're waiting, people start talking about gunshot wounds again but with less enthusiasm than before. When the on-call neurosurgeon eventually arrives he looks at the images with a detached air. 'No significant internal bleeding,' he says. 'No midline shift. No indication for surgery.' As if we didn't know this already. 'Get him to the neuro ITU and they can wake him up tomorrow and see how he is,' he says, and disappears.

'Is he going to die? I need to let them know if this is likely to be a murder investigation,' the policeman says.

'Probably not,' says the A & E consultant. 'Though God knows what kind of life he'll have.'

The anaesthetist wheels the patient off to the intensive care unit. The A & E team return to the department. We hand over to the evening team, exchange scrubs for civilian clothes and head out into the autumn dark. Tomorrow will bring what it brings.

As I sit on the train home, exhaustion descends. A mess of thoughts flit across my consciousness. How the man looked before we put him to sleep, his swollen eye, his moaning, the fact his left arm didn't move. I wonder who had pulled out the knife. I try to imagine what it must be like to be the perpetrator who did this to him. I hope they are able to wake the patient tomorrow and that he hasn't been left horrendously disabled. It's impossible to guess from what we've seen how he will emerge, and little that can be done to change it. I'm left with the conundrum of the patient's last coherent words rolling through my brain, as the train carriage rocks me to sleep: 'Sun, sun, sunny. Sun, sun, sunny.'

The Lady in the Bed

'I told you, you was stupid,' says the young man lying on the A & E couch, forgetting to wince for a moment.

'Why's that?' I foolishly take the bait.

'Cos you can't see the truth.'

'Which is?'

'That I'm fucking well dying and I need some morphine.'

'You're not dying.'

'How the fuck do you know? And anyway I'm in agony,' he continues, clutching his gym-sculpted stomach. 'And you can't tell me I'm not.'

'You're always in agony,' I say. 'According to your records, you've been attending all the emergency departments in the area in agony for weeks, and everywhere you go, every blood test and scan you get shows you're in good health. Morphine's not necessary, and it's addictive.'

'That's it?' he asks, incredulous.

'That's it,' I say. 'There's a waiting room full of people I need to see.'

Shaking his head and muttering, he pulls on his shirt, stands up and limps out, saying over his shoulder, 'I feel sorry for them. You're a shit doctor.'

'Another satisfied customer,' I say to myself, picking up the next canary-yellow patient card from a teetering pile.

'What did you say?'

I turn round to see Jasmine, one of the nurses, her auburn hair pulled back in a knot, staring at me as if I'm mad, a purple comma underneath each sceptical eye.

I shrug. 'Nothing. Three patients so far and nothing wrong with any of them.'

'Saturday night,' she says without pleasure, rushing on to the next task.

There are no windows in the A & E majors department, no seasons, no times of day, just strip lights pouring out a sickly bright light into the waiting room below. On a chair is a large grey slab of a man gritting his teeth in pain, sweating profusely. Two scantily clad women are dancing softly on the spot on either side of a woman whose head is thrust into a 'sick bowl'. A pair of standing policemen, thumbs tucked into the armpits of black stab vests, are joking with each other. Sitting between them is a huge man in handcuffs with an ink spider's web spreading up his red neck and face.

'Saturday night,' I say, even more depressed to be reminded of this fact.

Kevin——, 32-year-old male. Allergic reaction the next patient card states. Amazingly Kevin has talked his way into waiting in a cubicle (cubicles are gold dust in the department). Earlier this evening the handcuffed prisoner with the tattoo ripped its thick fabric curtain down and, as I approach, I'm confused to see a grey-haired woman in half-moon spectacles lying on the bed that dominates the narrow space.

'You're not Kevin,' I say as I enter.

'I am,' says a slim young man, sitting on a chair to one side. He has a remarkably unlined face for his thirty-two years, white skin, guileless hazel eyes, and full rosebud lips.

'Who's the patient?' I ask jovially.

With an air of modesty Kevin points at himself.

I squeeze into the cubicle on the other side of the bed. 'And who are you?' I ask the woman in the bed.

'I'm his mother,' she says grandly. 'I too have many problems . . .'

'I'm sorry to hear that,' I say, hastily cutting her off and waving the canary-coloured card, 'but Kevin is the patient today.'

Let's make this quick, I think. If we have to do two consultations for the price of one, this night will never end.

'So, Kevin, why are you here?'

He takes a deep breath. 'It all started earlier today . . .' he says with an air of mystery.

'Yesterday evening,' the grey-haired woman cuts in, indicating the clock on the wall, which shows the time is two in the morning. 'Or years ago, depending on how you look at it.'

'Let's stick with yesterday,' I say, pointing through where the curtain should be in the direction of the waiting room. 'It's busy out there.'

Kevin nods dutifully and takes another deep breath. 'Yesterday evening I had to go and collect my mum's cat from the vet.'

'Kevin's always had a soft spot for animals,' the lady pipes up from the bed. 'Takes after his mother in that way.'

'He's been unwell for months. But the vet doesn't think much is wrong,' Kevin continues.

The lady in the bed shakes her head in disbelief. 'It doesn't matter how many times we take him there. You wonder what they teach them at vet school.'

'I'm sorry to hear that,' I say, 'but I think we should skip the cat for now.'

The lady draws herself up in the bed. 'You can't hope to understand what's happened to Kevin without hearing about the cat,' she says. 'He's very unwell, problems with his guts.'

'Kevin?' I ask.

'At the moment I'm talking about Ronnie,' she says. 'Ronnie is important too.'

I look around the cubicle. 'And Ronnie is?'

'In a cage in the car,' says the lady.

Nothing surprises me any more. They have waited four hours in the middle of the night to tell me about their cat's health.

'OK,' I say. 'I'm struggling to see the relevance of this. Are you allergic to cats, Kevin?'

He looks horrified. 'God, no,' he says.

'I can confirm,' his mother states acidly, 'that Kevin is extremely fond of cats.'

I hold my hands up in surrender. 'Please tell me what happened, Kevin, to make you come to hospital and what, medically speaking, I can do for you,' I say.

'So I had to collect the cat at about six p.m.,' says Kevin, unflustered. 'Mum was in no fit state. I argued with the vet but they wouldn't hold on to him. I think we need to find a new vet –'

I rotate my finger in a circular motion to try to speed things up.

'It was a nice day,' says Kevin. 'The cat was behind me on the back seat. I had the windows of the car down and there was a warm breeze coming in.'

Kevin is so hard to hurry in his storytelling, and I'm tired and have spent so much of the last four months in this tomb of an A & E department, that I drift into a reverie. I begin imagining the soft-scented breeze wafting through barley fields, high scudding clouds in a blue sky, the feel of the sun on skin . . . Then I catch sight of the prisoner with the tattoo on his neck in the waiting room trying to catch flies in his mouth. Around him people are clutching bellies and hearts. Some are standing, some are sitting, some are even lying on the floor – the double whammy of feeling lousy and having to wait glazing their eyes.

'Can we cut to the chase?' I say. 'There are lots of other patients . . .'

'At that moment an insect flew in the window,' says Kevin, looking at me dramatically, 'and went straight past my head.'

I look up because there's a buzzing sound coming from the ceiling; it's one of the strip lights that is flickering at high speed.

'I tried to swat the insect but I had to concentrate on driving. I could hear it flying around in the back seat. When I heard the buzzing get louder I knew it was coming closer to me. I began to sweat a lot.'

He pauses dramatically and looks at me to check my attention. I'm distracted, rocking on my heels, trying to maintain concentration. I drift back into my own thoughts. 'Listen to your patient,' goes the old medical saying. 'They are telling you what is wrong with them.'

'I was terrified . . .' Kevin says.

Getting no response from me, Kevin says a bit louder, 'I was terrified . . .'

'Yes,' I say.

'Because I'm extremely allergic –' he looks at me carefully and enunciates every syllable – 'to pretty much everything.'

Apart from cats, I'm ashamed to find myself thinking.

A voice from outside the cubicle says, 'Knock knock,' and Jasmine, the nurse, pretends to draw aside an imaginary curtain and pokes her head in the cubicle. She looks flustered with the chaos of a Saturday-night emergency department behind her: 'Any bloods?' she says in a harassed voice.

'No thanks,' I say, watching Kevin's face as I demote him. His placid smile doesn't flicker.

'OK,' she says, raising one eyebrow at me as if to say, 'As this case is clearly not an accident or emergency, could you kindly get on with it?'

'Thank you,' I say in response to this prompt, aware that I need to find the energy from somewhere to gain control of this consultation. The imaginary cubicle curtain is redrawn. 'So . . .' I say, pointing at the clock on the wall, 'eight hours ago you were driving in your car, an insect came in and it frightened you . . .'

'You'll be wondering what kind of insect it was,' he says, like a prompter helping out a struggling actor.

'No . . .' I say.

He turns to his mother, her sharp eyes glinting behind the spectacles, two recumbent half-moons.

'We've been discussing this,' she says. 'We're not quite sure. Maybe a wasp or a mosquito or a fly.'

'So you were in the car with Kevin?' I ask.

'No,' she says. 'He was on his own. As I was trying to tell you earlier, I have this problem with dizziness. I'm waiting to have a scan to see what's going on but, in the meantime, I can't do much.'

'What kind of insect do you think it was?' Kevin asks.

There's a pause before I realize the question has been addressed to me.

'Why are you asking me?' I say. 'I was here seeing patients.'

'I know that,' Kevin says, irritation showing through for the first time, 'but I thought you'd know what sort of insect could make this happen.'

'Make what happen?'

'The swelling,' he says, pointing to his face. He looks at me trustingly with his cornflower eyes as if he has told me his deepest secret.

'And the itch,' adds his mother. She looks very relaxed in this place full of drunks vomiting and people moaning in pain.

'Swelling,' I say, looking at Kevin's unswollen face. On it is an unfamiliar expression that I suddenly recognize as a tender optimism. He is very pleased to be here, very pleased to be talking to me. They both are.

'Knock, knock.' It's Jasmine back again. 'I was wondering if you'd nearly finished,' she says, her voice laced with sarcasm.

'Possibly,' I say.

'It's just we could do with the cubicle. There are other patients, who are . . . unwell,' she says.

'Oh really?' I say, not hiding my annoyance. It's not as if I can say what I'm thinking which is that I'm ninety-nine per cent sure this guy is completely fine but, since I don't understand why he's here, I don't even know what question I'm supposed to be answering. That and I don't want to miss a life-threatening rebound anaphylaxis. 'We're not quite finished,' I say instead.

Jasmine shakes her head and withdraws.

Invigorated by the exchange I take a deep breath. 'So you were bitten by an insect about eight hours ago and your face swelled up, and now it's not swollen and you're here . . .'

'Yes,' says Kevin. 'I pulled straight over and called 999. The ambulance took seven minutes. Not very quick.'

'Did you have your EpiPen on you? Did you give yourself a shot?'

'I don't have one.'

'How come?'

'My GP doesn't think I need one. I seem to have a rare sort of allergy; it doesn't fit the usual patterns.'

'No clear trigger, no clear symptoms,' I mutter.

'Doctor Smith just doesn't seem to understand,' says his mother, ignoring me. 'We've had to get used to her attitude.'

'I can well imagine,' I say, pleased to have another colleague onside, however distant and however likely to be tucked up in bed. 'And what happened when the ambulance crew arrived?'

He pauses, hurt at the recollection. 'They refused to give me a shot of adrenaline.'

I feign surprise. 'Why on earth not?'

'They said they couldn't see any swelling.'

I nod sagely and reel off the other likely symptoms of an allergic reaction, none of which he seems to have suffered. I scan the patient card. 'Your blood pressure, pulse and oxygen levels were OK when the crew found you, and when you arrived here –'

'Well, that's another problem,' says Kevin. 'The paramedics refused to bring me to hospital. Said there was nothing wrong with me. So I had to wait for Mum to come and pick me up to get here. And it's not as if she doesn't have problems of her own.'

'It's true,' says his mum. 'There's a lot going on at present, my ganglions, my dizziness, my zinc levels, which Doctor Smith refuses to check.'

I put my hand up. 'I really think today we must focus on Kevin.'

He looks at me with gratitude.

'Of course,' she says, unruffled. 'I can tell you afterwards.'

'Then the nurse at the front here wouldn't put me on the list . . .' Kevin continues, pointing in the direction of the triage station.

'People just don't understand,' says his mother.

At this moment I notice a fat, heavy bluebottle in the cubicle, battling gravity on small wings. I suddenly feel certain that if Kevin's mother sees it, or, worse still, if this insect settles on Kevin and somehow generates a reaction of any sort, or even the claim of one, we could be here until sunrise. I watch horrified as the bluebottle lazily bobs and weaves its way in front of a strip light.

I place the patient card on the bed between Kevin and his mother and ask them both to confirm the address on it. While they are focusing down I step towards the back wall and take a swat at the fly. Kevin's mother turns to me sharply. The fly lazily ducks the blow and manages to reach the sanctuary of the wall. I grab the patient card back from her. 'So, Kevin –' I look him straight in the eyes, his face implacably calm – 'why are you here?'

'I guess I wanted this incident marked down for Doctor

Smith, so she knows this stuff isn't just all in my head. It's incredibly frightening when something like this happens. These allergies are ruining my life; I'm not able to work because of this.'

A flame of anger flares in me but is quickly extinguished by a wave of depression on Kevin's behalf.

'Let me just quickly check you out,' I say in as neutral a tone as I can manage. I squeeze his hands, palpate his neck and jawline, ask him to open his mouth wide and say, 'Ahhh.' I listen to one breath on each lung. It takes fifteen seconds in total.

'Let me reassure you, Kevin. I think you are very well. You're the fittest person I've seen tonight. In fact, on these numbers –' I wave the canary-yellow patient card – 'you're fitter than I am. And there's no evidence that today you've suffered any sort of reaction at all.'

Kevin nods sagely.

'I think something's happened to make you incredibly anxious about having allergies, am I right?'

'I think you are right,' he says.

'I think it's even possible that your worry about the reactions is a bigger problem than the reactions themselves and I would urge you to discuss *this* with your GP, not view her as the enemy. There are things, types of counselling, that can help with that deep anxiety. What do you think?' I direct this at both Kevin and Kevin's mum.

'I think you're a very good doctor,' he says.

'And a very good listener,' she adds.

'I think you should both get home to bed,' I say.

'Before we go.' Kevin raises his hand. 'You said you were interested in my mother's condition.'

'There are a lot of people waiting,' I say.

'It won't take long,' says his mother. 'It all started with fits and seizures when I was in my twenties. The neurologist said he'd never seen anything like it. The council won't give me a blue badge any more, though.'

'I have to go,' I say, and walk out of the cubicle.

Kevin stands up and helps his mother who swings her legs off the edge of the bed in a sprightly fashion. The blue-bottle buzzes past Kevin's face and he gently flaps his hand to move it on.

His mother looks at me coldly. 'Oh, well, another time,' she says.

'Maybe Doctor Smith'll finally get you that allergy testing,' she says to Kevin.

I shake hands with them in silence and watch them trooping past the Saturday-night carnage hand in hand, back to Ronnie and his problematic guts. Cured of whatever ails them by their time in A & E.

'Enjoy that?' asks Jasmine.

'Jesus Christ,' I say. 'Poor sods.'

'Bloody timewasters,' she says, as she hustles the next in line into the cubicle.

In most shifts you seem to get a preponderance of a particular type of symptom – breathlessness or headache or chest pain – and out of the Saturday-night chaos a pattern seems to be emerging. Each time I'm done with the last patient I call the next one from the waiting room and each time they don't seem to have much physically wrong with them.

After Kevin comes John, nineteen years old. His ambulance card states he has back pain and has attended A & E twenty-five times in the last twelve months with the same symptoms. Every time he comes he is unable to walk – a red-flag symptom for a neurological emergency. Like many people suffering chronic ill health, he is training in one of the health professions. Over the years extensive investigation turns up nothing that explains the degree of pain. He has ended up on large quantities of opiates and other pain medications, often prescribed when he arrives at hospital, and that his GP subsequently tries to wean him off.

Once I have persuaded him that he can walk, I get the prisoner with the spider's-web tattoo, who, after drunkenly beating up his girlfriend and failing to outrun the police in his car, suddenly claimed he had terrible chest pain. When I tell him his blood tests and heart trace are all fine he gets agitated and rips down another cubicle curtain before being hustled out of the hospital by the police. Then I get Gwen, a middle-aged woman and A & E regular, whose left foot every couple of days or so goes into spasm so severe it needs to be massaged by a hospital consultant.

It's four a.m. now and I've been working for eight hours straight and still haven't taken a break or even remembered to have a drink of water. Despite our efforts, the waiting room is even more packed. The vomiting girl has a drip up, still flanked by her dancing partners who are now slumped and snoring in chairs. The grey-faced man is up on the surgical ward pumped full of morphine, waiting to see if his pancreas can hold out, and there's a fresh crop of glazed, pained, unhappy people staring at me every time I pass.

I pick up the next patient card and it immediately makes me suspicious. Frank's home address is in a county 300 miles

away, his GP's address is in a county 200 miles in the opposite direction. This means we cannot access any of his past
medical history. Why doesn't he want us to know his past
medical history? Could it be because he's crazy, and his previous doctors have known it?

Sudden-onset headache. Stiff neck, states the triage note.

These words are big red flags for a very serious, potentially fatal diagnosis: a burst artery in the brain. Big red flags
hanging out of an upstairs window fluttering in the breeze,
perhaps with a few spotlights on the ground shining up at
them.

I head to the waiting room. One of the girls has woken up
and resumed her dancing. There are four or five more drunks
vomiting into standard-issue cardboard tubs. I call Frank,
my patient. He is dressed in nurse's scrubs. He is wearing
aviator sunglasses and as I call his name he gets up from the
chair and seems to stagger as he does so. I comment on the
scrubs he is wearing and he says he has been working a shift
as a nurse in a private hospital.

As I help him walk to the cubicle my brain revs into gear.
Despite the seriousness of the potential diagnosis there
are warning lights flashing in my mind. First of all, there are
the far-flung addresses. Then if the triage nurses had really
thought this was a burst artery, they shouldn't have left him
waiting in the waiting room for four hours but should have
escalated to a doctor straight away. Then there's the fact that
the patient seems to be a health professional. Of course health
professionals can be unwell, but they're also over-represented
in the world of fabricated illness. Then there's the staggering
about, which looks a bit like a poor piece of amateur dramat-
ics. And then there's the fact that if I wanted to fake an illness

to get attention I might well choose a serious headache because of the subjectivity of the symptoms. Plus, I'm feeling exceptionally jaded because no patient on this never-ending shift has actually been unwell.

I sit Frank on the trolley and rush him through the history of his symptoms. The tiny part of me that thinks it could be a burst artery knows time could be of the essence.

He tells me he has never had headaches before. He suffered severe sudden-onset pain in the head late yesterday afternoon while he was working his nursing shift. He took some painkillers and tried to carry on, but then a few hours later the pain suddenly kicked in three-fold and made him nauseous and then vomit. Now it was extremely painful to move his neck and lights were way too bright for him, hence the sunglasses. Frank's history could have been lifted from a textbook article on subarachnoid haemorrhages, arterial bleeds in the brain from which one in two patients will die. It's worrying but also suspiciously neat. Real patients rarely present with everything wrapped up in a bow like this.

Some families tend towards these swollen bits of artery in the head so I ask him if anyone in his family has suffered from anything similar. Yes, an aunt of his had a bleed on the brain before, he reports.

OK, I think. He's ticking literally every box here. This doesn't seem right.

I rush through an examination of the nerves that control movement, vision, balance and sensation to see if there's any objective evidence of a brain bleed. Everything seems normal. Everything apart from his neck, which, when I try to bend it, seems genuinely stiff. This gives me pause for thought. I try to slow down and re-evaluate, but my brain says this is another malingerer. He could be faking the neck stiffness, I rationalize.

I step out of the cubicle to discuss the case with the consultant.

'I know this sounds crazy,' I say after I relay the pertinent information, which all points towards us placing the patient in the resuscitation room lying with his head at a thirty-degree angle to the horizontal (to optimize the pressure within the skull) and getting an immediate CT scan of his head. 'But there's something about this guy, the addresses, the textbook symptoms, the way he's dressed. I just don't buy it.'

In my mind I'm pretty convinced he doesn't need the head scan. He doesn't need the radiation just to see the inside of a perfectly normal head. And then, when the scan is normal, he'll have to come in and have a lumbar puncture from the medics just to make sure there hasn't been a bleed, and use up a valuable hospital bed in doing so. And, above all, these people don't need to be encouraged by us falling for it. They'll keep coming back, clogging up this emergency department, when what they really need is a course of therapy from a clinical psychologist. Meanwhile people with problems that we can actually help with have to wait.

'No one I've seen tonight has been unwell,' I say weakly.

The consultant is one of the kindest doctors I've ever worked with. She smiles trustingly at me. 'You could be right, Tom,' she says, 'but we have to do the scan just in case.'

'Of course,' I say, feeling utterly defeated. And she's right. How could we not do the scan? That's why Frank has listed these very symptoms.

I book an urgent head scan, take a blood sample from the nurse, explain to him what we're doing and move on to the next patient. I decide that it's already so close to the end of the shift that I may as well just take my break at the end by leaving early.

I am relieved to find the next patient is manifestly unwell: feverish, coughing up phlegm, working hard at their breathing. The kind of thing I trained as a doctor to deal with. I've completely forgotten about the CT scan when Jasmine, the nurse, comes up to me.

'Well done,' she says, looking genuinely impressed.

'What?' I say.

'It's a subarach. You called it. We're bringing him back to resus.'

I feel sick to my stomach, as if I've just tried to kill a man. A wave of nausea rushes through me, a spurt of adrenaline. I get a beaker of water from the fountain and drain it. Stare up at the buzzing lights on the ceiling. I have another two beakers of water. I get a grip. I bleep the neurosurgeons and while I'm waiting for them to call back I bring up the head scan on the computer and scroll through images of the inside of Frank's head. There is a white blob right in the middle of his brain tissue showing the bleed that might kill him. When I speak to the neurosurgeons I harangue them to come and see the patient. I spend an exaggerated amount of time making sure the nurse gets the medication that will stabilize his blood vessels, that he gets propped up in the resus bed at the right angle and gets some decent pain relief. I fuss around him.

'Are you feeling OK?' I say to him, thinking this whole situation must be even more scary for him as a medical professional. He knows the physiology of what might happen. If the arterial bleeding persists his brain will start to get squished against the inside of his skull leading to almost certain disability or death. And he knows the odds: a decent chance he'll be dead in the next few days; a coin's toss that he will be alive in a year's time.

'I'm OK,' he says, keeping very still, trying to keep calm.

'You'll be all right,' I say, putting a hand on his shoulder. 'You're in the right place; we'll look after you.'

My stomach churns as I say these words and I wonder if, left to my own devices, I would have turned him away.

'Thank you for helping me,' he says. 'You took me seriously. You're a really good doctor.'

A few months later, on a sunny mid-morning, wearing civilian clothes on a day off, feeling relaxed, well rested, well fed and clutching a coffee, I wander into one of the hospital offices and log on to a hospital computer to follow up some of the patients I have seen. I feel butterflies in my stomach as I type in Frank's details. On the clinical software at this hospital the font in which the patient's name is written becomes bold if they have died. I am immediately relieved to see that Frank's name is written in normal type – the font of life. I press some buttons and find a discharge letter and then a follow-up letter from a neurology clinic. He spent several weeks in intensive care, had a tiny coil inserted via a blood vessel in the groin up into the aneurysmal section of artery in the brain to stabilize it and was discharged without mental or physical disability. The more recent clinic letter tersely states that he is 'in a good frame of mind' given what has happened and 'is realistic about the future'. So far the coin toss has landed heads you win for Frank. But he will almost certainly have been left a man who views his own brain as a time bomb.

Kevin, on the other hand, has been back to A & E twice in the intervening period. From the discharge letters it is not clear why.

Joker

The laughter greets us as we stand on the threshold of the bay to the rehabilitation ward and the sprightly consultant neurologist holds up her hand. 'Listen.'

The four of us stop and focus on the sound emanating from the bay. It is persistent, full-bellied and rich. There is something eerie about listening to this disembodied laughter. For one thing it's going on too long. Are we in on the joke or not? Outside the curtain we start laughing nervously.

'So I want someone to try a full neurology examination on this patient, and I want you all to try to work out what is going on with him,' says Dr Patel.

Joseph looks at the floor, Padme looks at the ceiling, I look out of the window. It has started to rain. We are at the height of the crowns of the chestnut trees lining the street and the raindrops are bouncing off the spring blossom.

'Oh, come on,' she says. 'Don't make me pick someone. The others will get something even worse to do.'

I glance in her direction, doing my best not to meet her eye.

'Excellent,' she stares at me. 'Tom, you do the examination.' Then she grins at the other two. 'And you both need to think of your best joke.'

Our surprise registers. 'I'm deadly serious,' she says. 'Your best joke.'

Dr Patel walks into the bay, and we follow, like goslings,

in our white coats. The laughter has stopped. One bed has the blue fabric curtain drawn round it. Surprisingly, given how crowded the rest of the ward is, the other three beds in the bay are empty.

Dr Patel speaks through the curtain. 'Sonny, are you decent?'

'I'm decent,' roars the disembodied voice. 'And of Scottish descent. But I don't resent, and I don't repent. Ha, ha, ha, ha.'

Dr Patel cocks her head on one side and gives us a knowing look. 'I've got some medical students to see you.'

'Students, stew, beef stew, atishoo. Bless you. Ha, ha, ha, ha.'

That rich laughter again. All gravy.

Dr Patel pulls the curtain aside with a flourish.

The surprise is that there is only one person in there generating all that mirth on his own. Lying in bed in a pair of pyjamas is a plump ageless white man, dark stubble on his fat cheeks, purple lips, a neck as wide as his head and a mop of brown curly hair. He has a jovial expression on his face. He rubs his hands as he sees us and says in Scottish-accented English, 'Doctor Patel, so these are the stew-dents. Students of what? Students of life. Students of death. Ha, ha, ha, ha.' He seems genuinely amused by his own banter.

I grab the drug chart hanging from the end of the bed. He is on whopping doses of antipsychotic medicine, which often leads to significant weight gain. He looks vaguely familiar but I am unable to place him.

'What can I do for you, Doctor Patel?' he asks.

'I was wondering if . . .'

'Doctor Patel. Doctor Foster. Doctor Death. Doctor, doctor.'

'Sonny, please listen,' says Dr Patel.

'Who's there?' finishes Sonny.

'I was wondering if Tom here could ask you a few questions.'

'Tom who?' He turns his gaze on me. He has pale blue eyes. 'Tom, Tom the piper's son, stole a pig and away did run . . . How does the rest of it go?'

I put on a grin and – the rest of the rhyme running through my head – approach the bed from the favoured right-hand side of the patient. 'Hi, Sonny, could I examine you?'

'Ye can do what you like with me.'

I want to test the nerves that come from his brain stem. This examination starts with a question.

'First I want you to tell me whether you've noticed any difference in your sense of taste or smell?'

'Not really, but I can smell you from a mile off, you fucker,' he says jovially.

I smile involuntarily, but I feel a bit taken aback and even more so when Dr Patel steps in. 'Sonny, please refrain from using bad language.'

'Ah'll refrain. Ah'll even retrain mesel'.'

'Now, Sonny,' I say, 'I'd like you to keep your head still. Fix your eyes on my eyes and tell me when you see my finger waggling.'

I stare straight at his eyes. He has luxurious long eyelashes and flecks of caramel in his cornflower-blue irises. At the twelve o'clock position on his right eye the white has a red discolouration. I waggle a finger at the periphery of my vision and he acknowledges the waggle the first time, but by the time I've moved it to the opposite corner his attention has faded and he's reading my name badge with interest.

'Tom, Tom the piper's son, stole a pig and away did run. Ha, ha, ha, ha.'

'I'm sorry, Sonny,' I say. 'Could you just keep your eyes fixed on mine and tell me when you see my finger waggling?'

He briefly glances at my eyes but is unable or unwilling to engage with my attempts to assess his field of vision. I shoot a glance at Dr Patel. She waves a hand at me to get on with it. 'Sonny, please keep your head still, but follow my finger with your eyes.'

This task is also too much for him. As I pull my finger across his field of vision he turns his head to look at it, no matter how many times I re-explain things. He will not do as I ask, and as a result I am not testing the muscles and nerves I want to.

I work my way through the rest of the standard cranial nerves exam aware of Joseph and Padme's amusement behind me.

'Sonny, can you raise your eyebrows?'

He does so. 'Ooh, ducky,' he adds camply.

'Close your eyes tight shut and don't let me open them,' I say.

Obediently he closes his eyes, but when I place my thumb and forefinger on his eyebrows and cheeks to try to open them, he flinches and jerks his head back.

'I'm sorry, did that hurt?' I ask.

He shakes his head and looks confused. I'm taken aback by this strange reaction.

When I ask him to smile he does so.

'Laugh and the world laughs with you,' he says. 'Cry and you cry alone.' He guffaws at this but nobody joins in.

I ask him to tell me if he can feel me touching his face.

'Can you feel it, can you feel it, can you feel it?' he sings.

I ask him to stick out his tongue and say 'ahhh'.

'Ahhhh, diddums,' he says in a baby voice.

So far I haven't found anything wrong with his cranial nerves but he is definitely behaving oddly. I take the ophthalmoscope offered by Dr Patel. 'Sonny, to conclude the examination I'd like to have a look at the back of your eyes.'

Again Sonny physically flinches away from me and holds his right hand up in front of his face as if protecting himself from an imaginary blow.

'That's fine,' says Dr Patel. 'Skip that bit.'

Now I move on to examine his arms and legs. Despite Sonny struggling to concentrate on some of the commands, it becomes clear that his right arm is working fine, but that his left arm has some weakness at the wrist and elbow. I try to establish his reflexes by tapping at particular points with a tendon hammer but he grabs the hammer from me and begins to tap out a rhythm on the side of the bed.

'If I had a hammer,' says Sonny, 'I'd hammer in the morning . . .'

'That's OK, Sonny,' I say, trying to retrieve the hammer, but he pulls it away from me, turns it round in his hand and starts jabbing at my stomach with the sharp end.

Humorously he says, 'Ah'll cut ye, lad.'

I pull the hammer from his grasp. 'Do you want me to stop?' I ask.

He is deeply amused. 'Do you want to hear a joke about a building?' Sonny asks.

'OK,' I say.

'I'm still working on it,' he says, and bursts into guffaws of mirth.

Dr Patel steps in. 'That's enough examination, Tom.' She smiles reassuringly. 'And speaking of jokes, I thought we could pay Sonny back for his time by each telling him a joke.'

The atmosphere gets awkward again. We are used to practising our examinations on patients but telling them jokes seems very odd.

Dr Patel points at Padme, who smiles nervously. This is her cue to tell a joke.

'OK, Sonny,' she says, moving to the side of the bed as I drop back. 'Why did the chicken cross the road?'

'I know,' says Sonny. 'To get to the other side.' He laughs uproariously at this.

'That's a good answer,' she says, 'but I was going to say, "To prove it wasn't a chicken".'

Sonny looks blankly at her.

We nod encouragingly.

'That's pretty good,' Dr Patel says, 'wouldn't you say so, Sonny?'

He shrugs, uninterested.

'OK, Joseph, your turn,' Dr Patel says.

Joseph approaches the bed. 'So, Sonny, a horse goes into a bar and the barman says, "Why the long face?"'

There is no flicker of recognition on Sonny's face. 'I don't get it,' he says.

'Tom?' says Dr Patel.

A joke I recently heard on the radio has got stuck in my head and the harder I try not to think about it, the more space it takes up there. I simply cannot think of anything else. I give up trying.

'It's a bit rude,' I say.

'I'm sure Sonny doesn't mind,' says Dr Patel, amused.

'OK,' I say. 'So, Sonny, a man goes into a job interview, and the interviewer says, "What do you think your biggest weakness is?" And the man says, "My biggest weakness? I guess that would be my honesty." And the boss says, "Well, I don't think you being honest around here is gonna be a problem . . ."'

I look at Sonny to see if he is following all this; he is looking at me and doesn't seem obviously distracted.

'And the man says, "Well, I don't give a fuck what you think."'

Joseph and Padme titter. Dr Patel is looking with interest at Sonny, who stares blankly. I probably rushed the punchline.

'You see the man was being honest, Sonny,' she says.

Sonny shakes his head in bemusement.

Dr Patel ushers us out of the cubicle. Behind us we hear Sonny laughing uproariously at something. When we are out of earshot Dr Patel gives us a shrewd look. 'So how do you feel?'

'Honestly?' Padme asks. 'Relieved to be away from him.'

We nod.

'He's incredibly wearing to be around,' Dr Patel agrees. 'Did you notice the empty beds around him? No one can bear to be in the bay for even half a day.' She suddenly frowns with sympathy. 'Poor man.'

She leads us into the empty family room where bad news is broken to patients and family members and we sit down round a small wooden table. She has an A4 piece of paper and quickly sketches a simple outline of a human brain.

'OK, Tom, so summarize your findings from the exam and anything else you noticed about Sonny. Then I'd like you to say where in the brain the lesion might be and what might have caused things.'

I've been anticipating this question since I started examining Sonny. I love neurology because of the way a patient's symptoms and signs applied to a knowledge of anatomy can give remarkably accurate locations of where the damaged bit of the nervous system is. It's the closest medicine comes to Sherlock Holmes. But it can be hard to think on your feet under pressure. Sometimes reciting the facts gives your brain the space to come up with the answer.

'So the cranial nerve exam was normal as far as I could tell. The upper limb exam showed weakness at the left elbow and wrist and possibly some spasticity. I was unable to test reflexes or his lower limbs.'

'Fine,' says Dr Patel. 'Can you summarize what else we found?'

'He has poor concentration on tasks. He tries to be funny a lot. But he isn't . . .' I trail off.

Dr Patel arches her eyebrows. 'Yes, do you know the name for that phenomenon?'

I shake my head.

'That's Witzelsucht,' she says.

'What?' we say.

'Witzelsucht.' She spells it for us. 'And now you've met Sonny you'll never forget it. It's German for joke addiction. So Sonny finds everything he says hilarious but he doesn't get a joke if someone else tells it. It's the result of damage to a particular area of the brain. Can you guess which bit?'

We look away from her, at the ceiling, the wall, out of the window, at which the wind is lashing the spring rain into drops that travel horizontally.

'He has also clearly lost self-control, hasn't he?' she prompts us. 'Which is managed from which bit of the brain?'

The frontal lobe, my own brain sings back. It's well named as it sits at the front of the brain, behind the eyes and fore-head. Every medical student is told about Phineas Gage, a reserved, devout nineteenth-century railway worker from America who got a one-metre metal spike through his frontal lobe and was transformed into a compulsive gambler and groper of women.

'The frontal lobe,' Joseph says.

'That's right,' says Dr Patel. 'So anyone want to hazard a guess as to what's happened to him?'

We look blankly into the distance, brains whirring. So Sonny has frontal lobe pathology, then there's the weak left hand, which equates to the right-sided parietal lobe, just behind the frontal lobe. He's young to have had a stroke and there's no history of slow progression to suggest a cancer or neurological disorder . . . And then it all floods into my brain and I feel the back of my neck tingling – the redness of the right eye, the flinch from my wanting to go anywhere near his eyes, the stabbing with the tendon hammer, and finally the realization that, underneath the layers of fat the antipsy-chotic medication that keeps him calm coats him in, under all that is a patient I've seen before.

I take the biro and on the sketch of the brain on the table I draw a crude knife entering above his right eye. 'Was he stabbed last autumn?'

Dr Patel looks at me sharply. 'Have you seen his notes?'

'No,' I say. 'I saw him when he came in to A & E.'

And I remember the policeman holding the plastic bag with the bent knife inside. And I remember how much that hour affected me at the time and how I'd hardly thought of it since, how it had been flooded under the tide of everything else that had been going on in my life. I realize that it has changed this man's existence for ever, left him pretty much intolerable to be around. It is hard to imagine many worse fates. And what was the word he had been heard saying while lying in front of the garages with blood seeping out of his eye. A complete mystery at the time. *Oh yes, 'sun, sun, sunny'*, I think. Son, Son, Sonny.

Smile

Her brown skin is almost translucent, her veins giving it a bluish tinge. Her legs are ramrod straight and stiff, her arms rigidly bent, fists up in a boxer's defensive stance. She has a small faded tattoo of a red bird emerging from flames on her right shoulder. She has a glazed expression on her unlined face, her green eyes unblinking, and a small volume of saliva is dribbling out of the corner of her mouth.

'Hi, Kelly, my name is Doctor Templeton,' I say.

There is no response. I try to position myself more clearly in her field of vision; it's hard to work out where or what she can see.

'My name is Doctor Templeton,' I say. 'I'm here to help you.'

There is no response. Her eyes blink. That is the only movement I can see.

I know only two things about Kelly: one is that she has multiple sclerosis, the other is that her gastric tube has fallen out. I have no idea how she communicates normally, whether she can speak or hear or voluntarily move any of the muscles in her body. I have been asked to put the tube back in and get her on her way home.

'I like your tattoo,' I say, looming over her and peering into her vacant face. 'That's a phoenix, isn't it?'

She doesn't appear to register the comment or my presence. Her eyelids blink and her green eyes stare straight ahead.

'I'm going to try to insert the feeding tube back in your stomach, OK?' I say. 'If you feel any pain, please . . . let me know. If you're able to . . .'

I tail off as I see not a flicker of recognition at my words.

I turn to the nurse, Nina, who's in the cubicle with me and whisper to her. 'Can she communicate?'

'I dunno,' says Nina too loudly for my liking. 'She's just been sent here straight from A & E.'

Kelly has a thin hospital gown on which reaches down to her knees.

'We're going to have to pull your gown up, Kelly, to expose your belly, OK?' I say, to her still, impassive face. There is no response at all. Nina brings the bedsheet up to cover Kelly's lower half and I pull the robe up to just below her breasts.

It seems the multiple sclerosis has not only made her muscles seize up into this awkward posture but has also made it impossible for her to swallow, hence the need for a tube directly into her stomach to feed her and give her medication. A hole has been punched from her stomach, out through the stomach wall and then through the abdominal wall, and a tube passed through to the outside world. For some reason this has come loose and fallen out.

We can see a small pink coin-sized hole on the upper left side of her abdomen. In theory I just need to poke a new tube back in, and quickly before the tunnel leading into the stomach closes up. But it's important I get the tube in the stomach and not into the abdominal cavity where it could cause severe infection. It's vital everything stays sterile as I reinsert the tube.

I clean the site around the hole and lubricate the tip of the new tube. With a gloved hand I try to stretch open the small hole just beneath her ribcage on the left-hand side of her abdomen so that I can insert the tube. There is a small leak of fluid from the external hole as I do so. The fluid worries me.

And as I'm fiddling with Kelly's tummy, gloved hands slipping on the slick of lubricant and abdominal fluid, I think back to a lecture from medical school.

Alexis St Martin was a young beaver trapper in his twenties who was shot in the stomach when a musket accidentally discharged at a trading post in the wilds of nineteenth-century Canada. He was treated by an army surgeon called William Beaumont who did not expect him to survive. Some ribs and a portion of lung had been blasted away and there was a hole the size of a forefinger into his stomach out of which poured anything he ate or drank. After a few weeks of this Beaumont managed to devise a system of dressings to keep in the stomach contents. Eventually, as the musket wound cured, an internal flap of flesh developed that meant the food stayed inside and his digestive tract began to function. The edges of the stomach and abdominal wall fused together but the wound never closed over externally, so there was a tunnel left from the stomach to the outside world, and the internal flap of skin could be moved out of the way with a finger.

Beaumont realized he had a unique opportunity to study the workings of the human stomach so he hired the trapper as a servant and, in between making him fetch water and cut wood, he experimented on him by placing small bags of food through the tract and into the stomach cavity. By this method the surgeon made some original observations about the process of digestion and the pH of the stomach juices, which, the same lecturer told us, is almost as acidic as battery acid.

I wipe the fluid away from the external hole in Kelly's abdomen with a sterile swab, worried it might burn her. And now I'm wondering whether the acid is leaking inside her abdominal cavity. Can the opening withstand this?

'Are you all right, Kelly?' I ask, glancing up at her face for signs of pain. She remains impassive and though I think I can see a single tear forming at the corner of one blinking eye I get no further response so I return to the task at hand. I ask Nina to move the light to give me a better look. I try to move the skin of the abdomen around so that we can scan the stomach beneath for its aperture but my gloved fingers are wet and slippery and the skin is pretty immobile, and all I can see is pinkness. I grip the skin tightly between thumb and forefinger but it slips from my grasp and pings back into place fiercely. I look at Kelly's face; it is entirely unmoved by the manipulation. She could be oblivious, I think hopefully, or then again she could be in excruciating pain and unable to express it. And how am I to know which?

Dim memories filter back of the long fasts and the indignity and pain Alexis St Martin suffered during Beaumont's experiments. Eventually, and much to Beaumont's regret, he ran off home. Beaumont pursued him in vain for many years afterwards, and when St Martin died his family decided to let his body decompose a while before burying him in order to make it harder for the medical profession to pursue him for further experimentation.

I change tack, pick up the short latex tube and gently start poking around in the hole, hoping by dumb luck to find the way into the stomach. After several minutes I've had no joy.

I can't get the tip more than a centimetre in, but I don't want
to push too hard or I might burst the tract and puncture her
abdominal cavity. I try to remember my anatomy lectures
and the various organs and blood vessels that may be in the
vicinity that could be threatened by my exertions. I'm beginning to lose my confidence. I'm sweating, and internally
cursing being given a job for which I have little training and
no experience. Then, just as I think I need to give up and
find a senior colleague, the resistance disappears and the
tube dives deep inside Kelly.

There is a deflated balloon around the tip of the tube which
I am hoping is inside Kelly's stomach. With my free hand I
grab the syringe of saline, which is ready and waiting, and try
to attach it to the valve that inflates the balloon. I clearly don't
lock it in place properly because when I depress the end of the
syringe saline liquid squirts all over Kelly's abdomen.

'Damn it,' I say. I turn to Nina who is unable to keep a
sceptical look from her face. She clearly thinks I don't know
what I'm doing.

'I'll get you another,' she says, and bustles off.

'Not quite there yet,' I say to Kelly, looking back up at her
face, which remains unmoving.

I focus on keeping the tube in exactly the same place in
her innards. When Nina returns with the syringe and plenty
more swabs I wipe up the saline that has gone everywhere
and manage to attach the syringe to the valve and squeeze
the saline into the balloon inside Kelly. When I gently tug on
the tube the balloon stops it from exiting the hole and causes
a bulge in her abdominal wall. I attach an empty syringe to
the tube itself and extract a tiny amount of colourless
liquid.

Nina rips off a piece of lemon-yellow litmus paper and places it in a kidney dish. I squirt a drop of fluid from Kelly's insides on to it. It quickly turns red, the pH of battery acid.

'Good,' I say, trying to mask my relief and project a composure I definitely don't feel.

I attach the external fixer to the tube, locking it in place.

'All done,' I say to Kelly, clearing away the gear. I walk back up the bed to get in Kelly's line of sight. 'I hope that wasn't painful,' I say. 'The tube's back in and in the right place, so we should be able to get you home.'

Her face remains impassive. She stares straight ahead with her eyes wide open. Her arms are still up in their boxer's stance, legs rigidly straight.

I look at her chest; she seems to be breathing shallowly and a bit quickly. I time her breathing with my watch. It is quick. *Is this because of the pain?* I wonder.

'Have we done obs on Kelly?' I ask Nina as she comes back into the cubicle.

'We were just supposed to get the tube back in and get her home,' she says irritably. There's a ward full of patients and a ward sister on her back.

'She's breathing a bit quickly, let's do obs.'

I take a stethoscope and listen carefully to her chest. I can hear fine crackles at the base of the right lung. Nina puts the thermometer in her ear and finds her temperature is raised. I order a chest X-ray at the bedside, and when it is done half an hour later I can see the fluffy signs of infection in her right lung.

I come back to the bed and loom over Kelly so I am in her line of sight.

'You've got an infection of the right lung, Kelly. We can

give you antibiotics for it. The consultant thinks we should keep you in for a night at least, then hopefully we can get you home and finish the antibiotic course through the gastric tube.'

She is on her back, limbs in the same stiff boxer's pose; there is not a flicker of recognition at what I'm saying.

'All right,' I say, 'I'll see you later.'

I turn to go when I notice a short young black man standing at the curtain. He is wearing a fire brigade T-shirt, his hair is braided into dreadlocks.

'Knock, knock,' he says, holding a hand up in greeting to me. 'I'm Kelly's brother. I came here as quick as I could.'

He waves over at the patient in the bed, grinning. 'Hi, sis. You been causing trouble again?'

I turn to look at Kelly. A broad smile lights up her face.

Gash

The push of a button flashes Luis's name up in the waiting room and thirty seconds later the door opens to reveal a short fit-looking man. His curly black hair is cut razor short at the back and sides like a footballer and he has a trimmed black beard. He is dapper too in a checked blazer, skinny jeans and cowboy boots. A pale blue bandana tied round his neck completes the cowboy image. He has a haunted look on his youthful face and a jumpy, restless demeanour.

Before he has even sat down he says, 'I tried to kill myself,' in English with a Hispanic accent. 'My girlfriend told me to come; she wanted me to get this checked out.' He unties the bandana and tilts his head back for my inspection.

I lean forward to look. There is a deep purple perpendicular bruise running round his neck. To one side the bruise narrows and becomes a gash in the skin. The wound is not that deep, but the edges are a centimetre apart at the widest and beginning to granulate. Between them is pink flesh with clear orange fluid weeping from it. *Lucky not to have hit an artery*, I think.

'It's too late for stitches,' I say. 'We need to put a dressing on and let the wound heal by itself. You'll probably be left with a scar. I assume you're able to swallow OK?'

He nods.

So much for the wound, I think, *but what about the mind attached to it?* The recklessness of his injury makes me worried for this man's safety.

I peruse the uncovered bits of his flesh – his arms – but there are no scars elsewhere, though there is the faintest of scratches on his wrist.

'How did it happen?' I ask.

A guilty look flashes on to his tanned face, then tears well in his eyes.

'I'm sorry,' I say, offering tissues. 'Why did it happen?'

We sit in silence for a while. The clock ticks, outside the city traffic hums faintly. The drunks in the park roar with laughter. Luis looks straight ahead of him at the opposite wall, which has a photo of a young member of a rainforest tribe: grass skirt, facial markings and chunky ear adornments. The expression on the youth's face is full of meaning but hard to read. Sometimes I think he looks confident, sometimes lost.

Eventually Luis speaks. 'Problems with my ex.'

'I'm sorry,' I say.

He nods and tears well up again.

I'm running late in clinic and part of me wants to hustle this consultation along, keep it lean, tick the boxes and get on to the next patient, but I know the only way I can help this man is to understand why he did what he did.

'Is this the girlfriend who brought you today?' I ask.

'No,' he says, and a grin briefly flashes on to his face.

Something about this grin, this acknowledgement of the humour in the dark reminds me of an old, close friend, some- one with whom I've lost touch. I try to focus on Luis.

'It's a long story,' he says.

'We have time,' I say, pushing the packed waiting room to the back of my mind.

The grin is quickly replaced by a hurt, raw look, some- thing closer to the emotional state he is currently in. He focuses his gaze on the tribal youth opposite him and tells me his tale, occasionally glancing up at me to check I'm onside with what he says.

Luis's 'long story' goes back two days. Life was going well. He loved his job in a firm of industrial electricians. Outside work he always hung out with his mate, Alejandro. The pair are from Colombia. They played football, drove around in convertible cars, hung out at bars and clubs, laughed and joked together, helped each other pick up women. When Luis needed refuge from his relentless social life he had a small flat that he could retreat to.

The only confounding factor in this set-up was his relationship with Gloria. She was also from Colombia and often hung out with the men. Together the trio had acquired the predictable nickname 'the three amigos'. But Gloria and Luis had also been seeing each other on and off for several years. She was beautiful, no doubt about that, but she was also volatile. Loving and wanting him close at one moment, argumentative and pushing him away at another, crazy jealous the next. He had realized over the years that they would never work as a couple but they were still friends and relied on each other and sometimes slept together. Her mother had come to live with her and Luis hung out at their flat regularly, helping them out around the house and being fed in return. This family-like set-up made him, thousands of miles from home, feel secure. But sometimes Gloria would just suddenly cut him out of their lives almost to spite him. She was like that, her mood swinging wildly. Usually, regardless of this, Luis and Gloria texted every day but last week, unaccountably, she had gone silent.

Then on the Saturday, two days before he is sitting in my

consultation room, Luis was sitting in his flat in his usual pre-night-out routine, radio playing dance tunes, looking at car stereos on his laptop, ironed shirt hanging on a small washing line, communicating with his friends by WhatsApp, when a message arrived from Gloria.

L u there?
Hi G
I need to tell u something.
What's up?

Then there was a pause. Luis could see that she was typing but it didn't arrive for a while and when it did it was short.

I'm seeing someone.

That hurt and triggered a pain Luis felt in his chest, but he could cope. Then he saw that she was still typing and the bombshell dropped.

It's Alejandro.

'I thought I was having a heart attack,' he says, still visibly shaken. 'I felt my head was going to explode; my vision went.'

'Why did it affect you so badly? She wasn't your girlfriend.'

He shakes his head. 'Alejandro, Alejandro is . . . a complete *puto*.'

'Huh?'

'*Puto*. He's a . . . a slut. He sleeps with anything that moves.'

'Oh right,' I say.

'I couldn't bear the thought of him with her. I know how

he treats the women he's with; he's always showing off about it.'

'So how did you get the gash?' I ask.

He wasn't drunk or high, but still it's all a bit of a blur. The thought of Alejandro with Gloria was unbearable, terminal; it felt like a brain tumour. Luis's first instinct was to message Gloria straight back. He was blunt and to the point: Alejandro is a *puto*, probably riddled with venereal disease, not worthy to lick her boots, she is killing him with this decision, can they meet and talk about it?

She was equally clear. She can get together with whoever she likes. She can look after herself. She is not Luis's property. She is sorry it's upset him, but he needs to man up.

This answer was unacceptable to Luis; it was as if it drove him crazy. He kept on at her via the small boxes on the phone. *She can't . . . She mustn't . . . She is killing him . . . What about her mother . . .* He almost wrote 'their mother'. Whenever another text box with rounded corners licked up on to the screen his heart started racing but the words they contained were always crushing.

Why are you being like this?

She didn't answer. He imagined his slut of a friend groping her while she was writing on her phone. This cranked his jealousy up another level.

Are you with Alejandro at the moment?

And then she went silent and he was left with the radio blaring tunes in his flat, alone in his suddenly ruined world. Now he really felt her out of reach, and his imagination went into overdrive. He proceeded from hectoring to threats. Not at her but at himself. I can't live with this. I'm going to kill myself, he wrote.

This brought her back, online at least. She told him not to be stupid, not to do this to her.

Luis reverted to his hectoring but she was unyielding. So he commentated via the text boxes as he unhooked the washing line. I'm going to hang myself, he wrote.

No reply. No text box. He sent the same message by email. But nothing appeared on either screen.

Luis waited for what felt like a minute. *Nada*.

He tied the washing line to a skylight handle, made a loop for his neck and, standing on the floor, pulled the noose tight. He thought he was going to faint but he didn't. Then he took a picture of himself and texted it to her.

I need help. I need an ambulance, he wrote. Nothing. No text boxes on the phone. The screen was blank. A deafening digital silence. He stood on the chair, watching the phone screen and the laptop, then looked at the skylight. Was this enough to kill him? He wasn't sure what he had intended but Gloria's silence, her callousness, when he had helped her so many times, made him suddenly adamant he wanted to die. He leaned into the noose, gradually taking the weight off his feet and the line pulled taut round his neck. He felt a searing pain and warm liquid on his neck. Part of the washing line's rubber coating had frayed away so it cut into the flesh. Suddenly the skylight fixing broke and he and the washing line fell to the ground.

He took another photo and sent it to Gloria by email and WhatsApp. Yet again there was no response from the machines. He got a pack of painkillers from the medicine cabinet. He swallowed all the pills with some water and in front of the unresponsive glare of the laptop lay down to meet his maker.

I look at Luis as he relates the story, distress still agitating him as he sits staring at the photo of the inscrutable young man from the rainforest.

'You thought the pills would kill you?' I ask, calculating that a smaller person might have stopped breathing.

'Yes,' he says grimly.

'You wanted to die?' I ask, wondering, as I ask the question, whether any of us really know what we want.

'Yes,' he says, tears falling again.

My mind whirls with statistics and with people I have known: young men, impulsive attempts and sometimes the irreversible tragic outcome.

'I'm sorry,' I say. 'And how do you feel now?'

'I don't know.'

The clock ticks on. I can hear the drunks get up and shuffle off up the street. Luis is making me nervous. Then he snaps out of his thoughts and continues his story.

Luis was surprised to find himself waking up. He felt woozy, and his neck was a throbbing agony that reminded him instantly that Gloria was seeing Alejandro. The bleeding had stopped. He had failed to kill himself. He checked the computer, and his phone. An hour had passed, and there was only one message, which was from Alejandro.

Leave Gloria alone.

The *puta*. She doesn't care. His mind was a whirlwind. He felt the only way to finish himself off was to cut his own neck

146

and he grabbed a kitchen knife but he couldn't bring himself to press home. He felt the walls of his flat closing in, being alone there suddenly felt unbearable. He remembered pacing around in confusion, unsure what to do. He considered trying to kill Alejandro, trying to get hold of more pills, booking a flight back to Colombia.

The plan that emerged was simpler. He found a bandage and a bandana and wrapped up his neck, put on his ironed shirt and headed out to the nightclub. There he fell to talking with another Colombian woman, Monica, someone he faintly knew, about his woes. He poured his heart out. She was shocked at the tale, at the gash, at his distress. He told Monica he couldn't bear to stay in his flat; it felt ruined for him. She said he should go home with her that night and sleep on the couch. He went home with her but didn't sleep. He couldn't get the slide show of Gloria and Alejandro together out of his head. His brain tortured him with pictures and dark thoughts all night.

Sunday was a nightmare of whirling emotions, redoubled efforts to re-establish contact with Gloria. But rather than generating sympathy his behaviour of the previous night seemed to have hardened her against him and he got no reply. He had lost her.

The thought of going back to the empty flat horrified him. Luis begged Monica to let him stay another night. She was what was standing between him and trying to kill himself again. She agreed, and the next day she drove him to his appointment at the surgery to get his neck looked at.

'And how are you feeling now?' I ask.

He shrugs. 'I'll be honest,' he says, 'I'm confused.'

'I'm not surprised,' I say. 'It must feel as if in one weekend you've lost your friend, your ex-girlfriend, your . . . sort of mother – your whole family over here in Britain – am I right?'

He nods.

'This is devastating for you,' I say, 'but you're going to get through it; you're going to repair things with your friends, and I'm here to help you.'

'Thank you,' he says, sounding unconvinced.

'Do you still want to kill yourself?' I ask.

He ponders this. 'Not at the moment. But when I think about going back to that flat, I wonder what I'll do.'

I look at Luis, smart footballer's haircut, a brain boiling with passion. A young impulsive man who is currently relying on a woman he met thirty-six hours ago in a nightclub for his security. We make a plan that involves him seeing the psychiatric team within the next few days, me in a week and the nurse now to dress his wound.

'Do you think she'll have me back?' Luis asks before he leaves. He looks like a lost child who needs comforting while the pain lasts.

'I've no doubt you'll be friends again,' I say. I shake his hand and clasp his shoulder, staring into his dark brown eyes. 'I'll see you in a week.'

When Luis walks back in a week later I feel a great sense of relief to see him. He is wearing a Stetson to go with cowboy boots and jeans, a clean red bandana tied round his neck. When he takes the hat off and rests it on his knees he looks pale, his face drawn, dark circles under his jittery eyes.

He undoes the bandana and I am pleased to see the gash on his neck doesn't look infected. There is some granulation inside the wound, which should just gradually rise up over time and fill the gap. At each end the wound is knitting together as if the edge of a smiling mouth were closing into an expression of perplexity. When he's retied the bandana I ask him how things are going. 'Not well,' he says, and stares resolutely at the photo of the face-painted youth in the rainforest.

'How did it go with the psychiatric team?' I say.

He shakes his head. 'I never heard from them.'

Damn it, I think. 'I'm sorry about that,' I say. 'That's no good.'

He waves my apology away. 'I think I know why,' he says.

It seems Luis had persisted with his barrage of electronic pleas to Gloria, all of which went unanswered. Desperately he sent her screenshots of previous communications he had had with Alejandro, which demonstrated his former friend's flippant and derisive attitude towards women. Soon after he realized that Gloria had blocked him from her messaging service and de-friended him from her social media account. He had been banished to the dark. Then came the blowback from his former amigo. Alejandro began goading him about his behaviour the previous weekend via text, calling him a *carechimba*, a *pendejo*, *hijueputa*, and telling him to stop dicking around. Luis threw his mobile phone in the river in frustration.

'So that's why the psychiatric team didn't get in touch,' I say.

Luis's nights were still a torment of nude images of Alejandro and Gloria together; his days a lament for the loss of his relationship with Gloria and her mother. Luis felt unable to face work because Alejandro was an employee in the same company. He had also stopped going out for fear of bumping into his ex-comrade. He was still staying with Monica, and had only nipped back to his own flat to get some things.

'I felt sick when I was there. It reminded me of the times me and Gloria were together.'

Luis was unsure for how much longer Monica would have him. He was sleeping on her couch, and it was a small flat.

He looks so lonely as he sits there hunched in on himself in the chair, staring at the rainforest youth with his make-up and earrings, the clock ticking away. *You've lost it all*, I think.

'Any further suicide attempts?' I ask.

'None,' he says, avoiding my gaze, 'but if I end up living in that flat I think I'll slit my wrists.'

I ask Luis more about his medical history to try to understand if there is a background mental health problem that can be addressed to help his current plight. But there is nothing to pin things on.

He says he was always a sensitive child who took criticism very much to heart. He is from a large family from a coastal city in Colombia and had a good relationship with his parents, both teachers, and his four sisters and two brothers. He has always been very close to his mother. No problems making friends or getting girlfriends. Not in trouble at school. Dabbled with drink and drugs but not in recent years. No previous mental or physical health problems. He is in touch with his family but hasn't felt able to tell them how he is feeling.

Luis is withdrawn, the adrenaline of last week's consultation a distant, sleep-deprived memory. Nine days in and the split from Gloria is taking on a permanent cast in his mind. He agrees that he should see the mental health team. I take his new mobile number. I prescribe him a short course of sleeping pills.

'Is there anything else I can do to help?' I ask.

'Get me Gloria back,' he says.

'You didn't have her before,' I say.

'I know,' he says, 'but I could have done.'

Still worried about the precariousness of his situation I arrange to see him a week later and tell him firmly he must seek immediate help if he starts feeling suicidal again.

When he walks in again, a grass-green bandana round his neck, Luis still looks pale, but he has more animation in his body, and his shy grin when I ask how he is doing makes me feel he might be turning a corner.

I undo the bandana. His neck wound is healing nicely. Red scar tissue is filling the gash. He's done a good job of keeping it clean. The perpendicular bruise has turned yellow.

He launches straight back into the events of the intervening days. He went and waited outside Gloria's place of work, a bank where she is a cashier, but then became scared of what she might say and fled, preferring the uncertainty to the possibility that she might reject him to his face.

He hasn't seen her since before this all happened. And he hasn't returned to work because he feels that if he sees Alejandro he will either attack him or freeze and be humiliated. Nor has he seen the mental health team. He forgot to return their call he says.

'Don't you want to see them?' I ask, worrying about being

the only doctor this risky young man has seen, wishing I had the backup of the specialists.

'I don't mind either way,' he says. 'Those pills helped a lot.'

'The sleeping pills?'

'Yes, it's amazing how a bit of sleep can help you think straight.'

'I'm glad,' I say.

'After a few nights' sleep I came up with a plan.'

'Excellent,' I say.

'A plan to get Gloria back.'

'Oh,' I say. 'OK.'

He decided he needed to get Gloria back via social media before risking a face-to-face meet-up. That she needed to be shown evidence of Alejandro's untrustworthiness in direct relation to her. To that end he set up a fake social media account in the name of 'Rosa', describing 'herself' in highly desirable and available terms, and copied pictures from a random Venezuelan woman's online profile, who he thought would be exactly Alejandro's type, and used these pictures on the account of his female avatar. He then dropped a note on Alejandro's account purporting to be from Rosa and they struck up a friendship. Alejandro entirely fulfilled Luis's expectations by coming after Rosa, '*como una perra en celo*'.

'What?'

'Like a dog on heat,' he says.

'Luis,' I say, 'do you think you're going to be thanked for all of this? Isn't it better to back off and for Gloria to discover for herself what kind of person this guy is?'

I look at him, his brown eyes sparkling between the dark circles. He's excited by his plan. He's doing something. He's working to get Gloria back. This is the second-best thing to having her back. Perhaps this is the therapy he needs.

'Too late,' he says. 'It's too late for that.'

It turns out Luis wasn't happy gathering digital evidence of Alejandro's intent and wanted to go further. To that end he asked a friend called Ana to help him out. She somewhat resembled the Venezuelan woman in Rosa's photos, though, he says, Ana was not from Venezuela, had different-coloured hair and was less thin.

'They all fake their pictures anyway –' he wags a censorious finger – 'and Alejandro wouldn't care.'

Luis had explained that he wanted Ana to pass herself off as Rosa, go to bed with Alejandro and surreptitiously film some of the action. He would provide the equipment.

'And Rosa agreed to this?' I ask, incredulous.

'Ana,' he corrects me.

'Right.'

'Of course,' he says, adding simply, 'I offered to pay her.

'I arranged for them to meet at a bowling alley on Saturday night, so I parked further up the street with a blonde wig and recording equipment for Ana and waited. I waited for a while and when she didn't turn up I texted her and she replied and said she couldn't make it.'

'Good,' I say.

Luis stares at me as if wondering whose side I'm on. 'I was sitting there, the rain coming down, with a blonde wig on the passenger seat, and I could see Alejandro pacing up and down under the lights of the bowling alley . . .'

I can see a vein in the neatly shaven side of his head pulsing at the memory. He clenches and unclenches his fist.

'This was the first time you'd seen him, since . . . ?'

He nods.

'How did you feel?'

'I felt . . . I felt *inflamado*. Inflamed? Is that it?' A jagged grin crosses his face and he turns away from the rainforest youth to me. 'For a moment I considered putting on the wig and marching up to Alejandro just to see what would happen.'

I stare at Luis. He grins at the lunacy of it all.

I believe he grins at the realization of how the strength of his belief and desire is forever crashing on the rocks of reality. But his belief and desire – whether described in terms of synaptic chemicals or love poetry – is the sea he is swimming in. This, now, is how he can be close to Gloria. Just as small boxes of text on an LCD screen had made him feel close to her before. Without his scheming, without holding on to this hope, he feels unbearably lonely.

'Christ,' I say, 'please let this be an end to it, Luis.'

'Am I crazy?' he says, suddenly serious.

'Just temporarily,' I say. 'We call it lovesickness.'

'*Enfermo de amor*,' he says, nodding, the grin vanished.

We devise a plan. A boring, practical, medical one. It involves exercise, getting back to work, talking therapy. The mental health team have spoken to him and classified him as low risk, offering him an appointment in two months. So I ask him to arrange to see me whenever he needs.

He comes in a few weeks later, looking a better colour, bouncier. A white bandana this time, wound granulating nicely up to skin level now, still pink. The exercise has helped with his mood, he says. He doesn't feel he needs the talking therapy, so he cancelled the appointment. He is still living with Monica.

'She's really looked out for you,' I say.

'She has,' he says. 'I still can't cope in my flat. It feels so empty.'

Luis is more concerned with what's been going on with Gloria. Apparently she re-friended him on the social media site and his immediate response was to send her his dossier on Alejandro's unconsummated manoeuvres with the fictitious Venezuelan. He didn't hear anything back from Gloria but a while later saw that he'd been de-friended by her again.

'What a surprise,' I say.

He throws me a devilish grin. 'I still think it was the right thing.'

He's still obsessed with Gloria and Alejandro being together, still dreaming about them.

'She wasn't even your girlfriend,' I say.

'I love her,' he says.

'Not enough to be with her,' I say.

It seems like her previous boyfriends had always been difficult for him to cope with, but it's the thought of Alejandro defiling her that cuts him in half.

'But it's OK,' he says. 'I have a plan.'

'Oh,' I say, 'another one.'

'This one will work.'

'That worries me,' I say.

'I'm going to hit Alejandro where it hurts.'

'No violence, please.'

'This isn't violence,' he says. 'I'm just going to poison him.'

'Luis, stop right there,' I say. 'I'm obliged to tell the police if you're planning something violent.'

'Not poison to kill, poison to . . . to take away his manhood.'

He pulls something out of his pocket. It's an amateurishly

put together sachet containing pink granules, with a series of words written in Spanish that I don't understand.

'I got it from a witch,' he says.

'A witch?' I say, holding out my hand for the sachet.

'Yes, a Colombian witch, a *bruja*. I got it online.'

'I see.'

'It's an elixir that makes a man *impotenti*.'

I hold the sachet. 'What do you mean impotent? For half an hour, three days, for ever?'

'The only problem is how to get Alejandro to take it.'

'That's not the only problem,' I say. 'The problem is you're obsessed, the problem is you're impatient, the problem is you've wasted your money on this rubbish. You just need to wait; Alejandro's going to self-destruct any moment. Don't give him this.'

Luis sits in his chair with the face of a naughty boy.

'A witch?' I say.

'I need the witch because you're not helping me,' he says eventually.

'I'm a doctor, not a hitman,' I say. 'I'm here to listen and advise, not resolve your relationship problems.'

'Yeah,' he says, putting his hand out for his sachet of impotence elixir.

'Why don't I keep it?' I say. 'Then you won't be tempted to give it to Alejandro. God knows what it's got in it.'

'That cost me a lot of money,' he says.

We talk for a long time. Eventually he relents and I put the sachet up on a shelf high above my desk.

A fortnight later I find that Luis is on my clinic list. My heart leaps, I'd neglected him. But when he walks into the room he looks better than I've seen him yet. Head held high. Full of energy. There's no bandana on his neck now, just a narrow pink scar.

'Good to see you,' I say, surprised by how much I mean it.

'*Lo mismo*,' he says. 'I'm feeling much better. You were right.'

'Great,' I say. 'Right about what?'

'Gloria said she would see me again,' he says with a big grin on his face.

I feel a massive sense of relief. 'Great,' I say again, and pat him on the shoulder.

And then he launches straight in to his story, how Gloria unblocked him on the messaging service and admitted she found Alejandro's behaviour troubling. She has agreed to meet Luis in the next few days with her mother. 'She misses you,' she'd said.

'I'm delighted to hear it,' I say, unable to suppress my pleasure.

We talk a bit about his getting back to work and trying to repair things with Alejandro at some point.

'I guess I won't need to come here so often,' he says. He points at the photo of the youth from the rainforest. 'I'll miss him, and you won't want to hear my stories any more,' he says with his shy boyish smile.

I laugh. 'Well, hopefully there won't be any wild stories to tell. I mean, things should settle down, right?'

'But you liked hearing them, I think?' He looks at me slyly.

I think about that for a second. There's something troubling me, but of course I answer positively. 'Sometimes you had me worried, but I suppose in a way I did.'

He looks at me seriously. 'It helped, you listening,' he says, 'being here for me. You didn't judge me.'

'I'm very glad things are better,' I say.

'I hope I haven't wasted your time,' he says.

I ponder that. What have we done here? Why did I see him so much? Was he ever a danger to himself? Looking at him now he seems pretty good. Not undamaged, but who of us are? On reflection, with hindsight, the whole escapade seems wildly eccentric but not dangerous. As if there has been something unmedical running through our relationship.

But that gash, the washing line, that was serious. And from experience you never know when the ripples from such acts, however much they seem to be settling, will coalesce back into a tidal wave.

'No,' I say indignantly, 'you haven't wasted my time. It was important that you came. And actually you could do me a favour.'

'For sure,' says Luis. 'Anything you want.'

'Will you phone up the talking therapy and give it a go?' I say.

Luis looks sceptical. 'Oh, that. I don't think I need that. What's it even about?'

'You talk they listen; they talk you listen. Just try it, I think it will help.'

He grins, and once again I see in him my old friend.

'I'll do it,' he says.

And then the obvious strikes me. We are similar ages. He lost his *amigos* just before he came to see me. And for my part he reminds me of an old friend and a type of friendship that I've also lost and that I miss. We've been hanging out.

'In fact,' I say, 'you've been helping me too.'

The drunks are chuckling on the bench outside my window; the clock ticks.

I pick the sachet of pink granules off the shelf above my desk. 'Do you want this back?' I ask.

Luis grins that boyish grin again and waves a hand, the wound on his wrist entirely healed. 'No need. You keep it, doc. Who knows when you might need it.'

I laugh and lob the sachet across the room and into the bin. 'So what are you thinking of saying to Gloria?'

Phoenix

The bleep in my pocket buzzes into life and the radio call from the operator intones, 'Adult crash call, Cedar Ward, Level 7.'

Damn, I think. It's just one floor up. I'll be the first there. I walk briskly along the corridors of the hospital, dark and silent apart from the hum of the generators and air con in the middle of the night. I take the stairs two at a time, muttering the stages of the life support protocol to myself like a prayer.

Cedar Ward is silent, the communal areas empty and lit only by a few lamps. A nurse darts out of the second bay so I head straight in. Three of the beds contain sleeping patients. The fourth is enclosed by a blue curtain through which lights gleam and activity can be heard.

I pull it aside to see a female nurse standing over the bed giving a body chest compressions. A healthcare assistant is at the head end, putting an oxygen mask over the patient's face. The patient is attached, via two pads stuck on her chest, to wires that terminate at a cardiac monitor and defibrillator. On the monitor the trace of the heart's electrical activity bounces with the chest compressions.

'What happened?' I ask.

'We just found her with no pulse,' says the nurse, puffing and panting with the exertion.

'Can you stop for a moment?' I say.

I come round past the nurse to assess the patient.

The patient is still. Her head is tilted back, the oxygen mask partially obscures her face but it is not misting with breath. I press her neck with my fingers feeling for a pulse, but all I get is my own pulse bouncing back. Now the chest compressions have stopped the heart trace on the monitor shows a single flat line.

'Back on the chest,' I say and the nurse beside me immediately responds, leaning over the patient and putting her full weight into pressing down on the patient then releasing, pressing then releasing.

Then I notice a faded tattoo of a red bird emerging from flames on the patient's coffee-coloured shoulder.

I pull the oxygen mask off. It's Kelly, the woman with multiple sclerosis and the feeding tube I saw a few months back.

'OK,' I say, trying to slow my whirling mind, 'I don't think she's for resuscitation.'

The nurse looks at me sideways.

'If I take over the chest compressions, can you go and check her notes for the purple form?'

The nurse steps away and I take over, pressing rapidly down on Kelly's breast bone then releasing to keep the blood in her body circulating.

'Are you sure?' she asks.

'A month ago she wasn't,' I say. 'Just please quickly check.'

The nurse nips out of the cubicle, and I keep compressing and releasing on Kelly's chest, during which time she shows no signs of life. Within thirty seconds the nurse is back waving a purple piece of paper. 'You're right,' she says.

I stop the compressions, wipe my brow and take the form from her.

'I'm just covering from another ward, that's why we didn't know,' the nurse says in justification. 'The nurse from this ward was unwell and had to go home.'

'Don't worry,' I say, 'you did the right thing. Please cancel the crash call and then phone her brother and let him know she's died.'

The nurse goes out of the cubicle and the healthcare assistant takes the chest pads off and switches off the defibrillator and the oxygen.

Polly, my medical night team colleague, comes racing into the cubicle. I shake my head at her. 'She's not for resus,' I say. 'It was a mistake.'

Polly looks at me carefully. 'You're sure?' she says, looking at Kelly thoughtfully. 'She looks so young.'

'Yes,' I say, pointing to the purple form. 'I know her. I can confirm the death.'

Everyone leaves me in the cubicle with the curtains drawn. A low light casts a shadow across Kelly's meagre body under the sheet.

I'm struck by how much stiller she looks than when I saw her a few months back, even though she scarcely moved a muscle then. Her face has the sunken, waxy quality even the recently dead get. Her eyelids are half closed. With some force I pull them open and shine a pen torch at the large black pupils underneath. They remain large and unmoving despite the light's glare.

I listen to her lungs and heart for a few minutes. No movement of air, no contraction of muscle. Just the sounds of the body settling chemically. After the chaos, the stillness. The gradual betrayal she experienced from her damaged body has been rendered irrelevant in death.

Kelly lets out a gasp and I flinch, but it's just her body settling.

The nurse comes back in and starts packing up the heart monitor.

'I saw her as an outpatient a few months ago,' I say. 'Do you know why she was in hospital?'

'Her notes say she came in a few days ago with a chest infection,' the nurse says.

A bleep calls me away and I come back later to fill out my notes and find Kelly's brother sitting in the armchair by her bed. Behind him a waxing crescent moon is visible in the night sky, which is a muddy brown above the lights of the provincial town. While I fill out the notes under a low yellow lamp we talk, with Kelly's still body between us.

Kelly's brother tells me how, when they were young kids, she used to dress him in girls' clothing because she wanted a younger sister. How she protected him from bullying at secondary school, how she bought him his first pop single and his first alcoholic drink. What an amazing dancer she was. Her great rip of a smile. How she was the bright one in the family, the first ever to go to university, how she helped him with his application for the fire service. How one Christmas she suddenly couldn't see properly out of one eye. How long it took to get a diagnosis. How she hid the rapid worsening of the illness from him for a long time. How upset she got as she started losing the use of her limbs. How furious he became at a world in which his sister could suffer and then suffer more, and then endlessly suffer more. How he went off the rails for a while at this time, and how she bullied him back on to them, and would say to him, 'Stop moaning. It's not happening to you, you bastard.'

He is looking at his dead sister throughout all this.

'I'm going to miss her,' he says, coming to a halt with his memories and staring out into the pre-dawn sky. He looks up at me. 'I just wish there was something that could have been done,' he says.

I mutter something about people working on new treatments but research being rather slow and there being no recent breakthroughs when he interrupts.

'No, I don't mean that. I mean, something to stop her suffering. She's been in such a bad way for so long. Would you doctors have been able to . . . to finish things earlier, back before it got worse?'

'Not in this country,' I say, beginning to understand what he means. 'They've talked about changing the law but currently we're not allowed to.'

'No, I don't mean the law. I mean, could you?' he perseveres. 'Do you have medicines that could do it?'

I'm stunned by the question. We spend half our time in hospital desperately struggling to keep people alive and trying not to harm them. Killing them would be, technically speaking, child's play.

'Yes, we could,' I say.

'It would have been kinder,' he says.

Through the glass of the window the brown night sky over the provincial city is lightening. Some of the windows of the houses begin to glow as people contemplate a new day.

The bleep in my pocket vibrates. *Adult crash call, Cypress Ward, Level 2.*

'I've got to go,' I say. And I leave Kelly and her brother alone together for the last time.

Middle Age

Labyrinth

It's mid-afternoon on a sultry summer day. The smell of die-
sel fumes, grilled meat and cannabis, the sound of creaking
bus brakes, R & B music and snatches of the Test match float
from cars and flats – there's a general holiday feel, people
shouting louder, trying to get business done a bit quicker.

The old psychiatric hospital has been in this suburb of the
vast, rambling city since Victorian times. Many of its buildings have been condemned and replaced over the years so
now it is a sprawling, incoherent, red-brick campus of the
troubled, the suffering, the stricken, the insane. From the
road it looks like a shabby university site completely devoid
of people. Look closer and you might notice the discreet bars
and shades on most of the windows.

A black cat stretches itself out on the windowsill by the
front door, licking its paws. Three of its feet are white, like
socks. It looks as if it has forgotten to put on the fourth. I
meet Abdul, the psychiatric registrar, in the lobby. The security guards slowly process our identification badges and get us
to sign a sheet of paper. They give us keys for lockers to put
our bags into.

Abdul has just got off the phone. A violent patient needs
urgent assessment. All we know is that she is a woman in her
forties, who had been hitchhiking. Something went wrong
and the police were called; when they tried to detain her she
started biting and punching them. Something about the

incident made the police detain her under the Mental Health Act Section 136. Now she is in a police van on her way to the '136 Suite', a safe, specialized area for acutely distressed patients, where she will be assessed and where we will decide whether to bring her into the hospital or let her go.

The 136 Suite is on the opposite side of the hospital. We have a brief discussion about which route to take. I favour walking round the outside of the hospital and getting some sun before we face this violent-sounding patient. Abdul decides we should take the most direct route through the middle of the hospital, passing through a series of wards.

We walk down a few corridors and get ourselves buzzed into the acute female ward. The patients are mostly in the shared lounge area. Several of them are pacing around or else standing swaying on the spot. They are mainly acutely psychotic or manic and on high doses of sedating meds. This leaves many of them restless, as if their chemically suppressed wild thoughts have to find an outlet. The television needs repairing. It was recently smashed by one of the patients who had become sick of being threatened by the world government through their agent, a famous daytime TV presenter.

This is where our 136 patient will be brought if we feel she has to stay. Abdul is asked to talk to one of the patients about being allowed out for a funeral. This is the risk of the direct route to the 136 Suite, all the other patients lie in our way and will slow us down.

Another of our patients, large and fierce and in the midst of a heavily tranquilized mania, is swaying from side to side.

'Who are you?' she says, reaching up to touch my face. 'What do you want?'

'You know me, Wendy,' I say. 'I'm just passing through.'

'But why don't you stay a while?'

'Things to do; people to see,' I say. 'We'll be back.'

'You don't really care about us, do you?' she says.

The 'really' makes it an even harder question to answer.

'Of course I do,' I say, but who am I saying it for?

Destiny lies on a sofa, arching her back and looking at us upside down with staring eyes. Even upside down she is beautiful. She is young and tormented by horrific persecutory delusions that mesh with the real-life problems she's been having with drug dealers and other people on her council estate over the past few years. Her waking hours are wracked by the clear belief that she will be – and that her family are currently being – subjected to torture by these people. When her parents come to visit, which is less and less often these days, she is always amazed to see them alive. It doesn't seem to matter how many times the reality is discussed with her, however much antipsychotic medication she is on, she still believes that this hideous situation is playing out. As a group of strangers who have detained her indefinitely on the grounds that she is mad, it's difficult for us to convince her that her detention isn't part of the plot against her, especially as she is surrounded by quite erratic people and is extremely distressed by the restrictions that we are placing on her.

Abdul has finished now. I look at Destiny's upside-down eyes, hold up a hand in defensive greeting and pass on through.

We walk down two more corridors. A locked door yields to the magnetic stripe of our security cards. And another locked door after that one. And then we are into the acute male ward. As we enter the main lounge, another patient I've come to know through my visits here leaps out of his chair and asks me what I think of Liverpool's new striker.

'It's cricket season, Marlon. I'll get back to football in August.'

'I don't know if I'll still be here in August,' says Marlon.

'Fair point. I'm pretty sure you'll be better by then,' I say. 'Is he any good?'

Eventually I extricate myself from the torrent of information about this incredible striker, Marlon's own astonishing football skills, his sexual prowess and then his sexual frustration in this unit. We write up some extra medication to help another patient – a man with psychosis and a personality disorder – to sleep. We share some banter with a few other patients and then we move on again.

We walk on through the ward and use our swipe cards to open two locked doors. We head on through a series of dark corridors before swiping open another locked door to enter the old-age psychiatric ward, hoping to quickly cut through.

We say hello to Moses, the lead nurse on the ward, a tired-looking man with dark-rimmed glasses pushed up on to the grey fuzz of his head.

'How're the kids, Moses?'

He massages his temples. 'A headache,' he says. 'But listen, guys, while you're here would you mind quickly assessing a new patient?'

Now the foolhardiness of our plan to take the direct route through the hospital really hits home. It's direct when measured out in metres, but psychologically we're veering all over the place, constantly losing our thread.

'We're in a rush,' Abdul says.

'I wouldn't ask,' says Moses, 'but we have another patient being brought in and I could really do with the assessment room.'

Abdul shrugs. Moses is a helpful nurse. The work needs to be done at some point anyway and perhaps the thought of the violent 136 patient at the other end of our journey makes us happier to pause for a while.

'Just a quick suicide risk,' says Moses. 'He might be able to go home,' he adds hopefully.

Earlier that day, Moses explains, Terry, a man in late middle age, had been found by his wife sitting in their car in their garage. A hose had been attached to the exhaust pipe and led in through one of the windows. The key was in the ignition but not turned on. His wife had shouted at him to get out. He didn't. But nor did he turn the key. His wife ran for the phone and called an ambulance. Then she returned to the garage to watch over him.

Terry stayed in the driver's seat, hand on the key. She rushed to let the paramedics in when they arrived. As they hurried into the garage he turned the ignition on. One of them opened the door and turned it off. They put him into the ambulance and brought him to the hospital. They removed his belt and laces, gave him a plastic beaker of water and put him in the interview room.

We unlock the door and walk into an anodyne grey-painted room with a screwed-down bench and table and two plastic chairs. Terry is sitting on the bench. He is still, impassive. He hardly turns as we come in through the door. He has pleasant features and a good head of wavy grey hair. Looks to be in his sixties. He is wearing a pair of faded jeans, a thick grey cotton shirt with streaks of green paint on it and desert boots with their tongues hanging out. When we introduce ourselves he turns and speaks quietly, calmly in a mild city accent. A very reasonable voice. I notice that he has dark brown, almost black, eyes.

My task now is to try to assess the seriousness of this attempt. Was it a coincidence that his wife had found him just before he switched on the ignition? Did he know that she'd be coming to the garage at some point, or was it his intention to die?

'Oh, I knew she was coming,' he says. 'I called out for her.'

'Why?'

He turns to us and a sly smile plays on his lips, as if he is reviewing a hilarious private joke. His eyes, though, remain unsmiling. 'I was just trying to scare her.'

There is a pause in the conversation while we wait to see if he means to continue, but Terry seems to think his explanation perfectly satisfactory. His smile disappears and he looks to be under some strain. Some distant cricket commentary flutters in through the window that has been opened to its maximum five centimetres. There's a sadism to Terry that makes me wonder less about his and more about his wife's safety.

'Why, Terry?'

He goes quiet. He looks as if he doesn't want to tell us what he thinks he knows. It's private. Why would he want to tell us, complete strangers? Why should he tell us? It's unspoken but he must know that we represent the power of detention in this mental hospital.

We wait. There is nothing else for it. You can't force people to talk. Not really. But how can you assess somebody's mental health if they don't?

'We really need to understand why you did what you did.'

Some sort of internal debate over, he looks off into the distance, steadfastly silent.

'Has your wife done something to annoy you?'

He laughs quietly, bitterly, to himself. Shaking his head as if to say you couldn't possibly understand.

'Have you been painting the house?' I ask, trying to get him talking.

'Lounge,' he says.

'Nice shade of green,' I say, pointing to a large paint streak on his sleeve.

'You like it?' he asks. 'It's called Enchanted Eden.'

'Do you have kids, Terry?'

'We've been married for forty years,' he says. 'No kids. At first I didn't want them. Then when I did, it didn't happen.' He lapses into silence again, as if he's been conned into giving too much away.

'Have you ever done anything like this before?'

He grimaces.

'Did something happen recently to make you do this?'

He shakes his head as though it will be hard to explain.

'We can't help you unless we understand what's going on, Terry.'

At first it isn't clear that he's even listening. There seems to be an internal struggle going on. Then he sighs long and deep, and turns his brown-black eyes to us.

'She had one boyfriend before me. Just one. I never knew his name, or anything much about him. This was back in the sixties. Who knows what they got up to . . .'

Excitement and cheering from the cricket commentary wafts in the window on the warm breeze.

'It's hard to talk about.'

'You're doing a good job,' I say.

'A few years ago I was in the garden, out the back of the house, when a man came to the door and my wife answered. She seemed to spend a long time at the front door talking to him but eventually he went away.' He turns and fixes us with his gaze. 'I didn't get a good look at him, but I noticed the car driving away was a silver hatchback. And I suddenly realized that this was the old boyfriend.'

'Realized how?'

'I asked her straight out, later that day . . .'

He looks at the floor, disappointed. 'She denied it. Said it was a travelling salesman. But of course she would say that kind of thing. Then we began to get the phone calls . . .' He trails off.

'What phone calls were those, Terry?'

'Oh, just once or twice a week. When she picked up the phone she'd pretend it was someone selling something. But I knew it was him.'

'What about when you picked up the phone, Terry?'

'She's the one who answers the phone; I never got him.'

'What did you think was happening?'

He studies the back of his hands, Enchanted Eden on his nails. 'I knew what was happening. They'd started again.'

'Again?'

'Just like back then.'

'That's a long time ago,' I say.

'Yes,' he says.

'How did you know?'

'Oh . . . I just knew. When you know someone that well you can just tell.'

I look at him wondering. He's right that we can intuitively tell a lot about people from their 'non-verbal activity', but his intuitions seem overconfident.

'Had you ever met the man before?'

'No, but she's my wife.' He can tell I'm sceptical. 'I know her.'

'Did you discuss this with her? Ask if anything was going on?'

'Of course, and of course she denied it.' He stares at us shrewdly with his dark eyes. 'I don't blame her for that.'

It looks as if he's wondering whether to share his next secret. He seems to decide that he needs to say more to convince us of his sanity. 'So I came up with a plan. I needed to confront him, but I didn't know where he lived so I started driving around looking for silver hatchbacks. If they were parked by a house, I'd knock on the door.'

I look at him blankly. There must be thousands of silver hatchbacks in this part of the city, and no reason to think this man lives nearby.

'You see I'd heard the voice at the doorstep two years ago. I knew I'd never forget it.'

'Do you realize how this sounds?' I say. What Terry is telling us makes me think that he is crazy, that he almost certainly has pathological jealousy, the so-called Othello syndrome.

We sit in silence. We all spend time in the grey borderlands between madness and sanity: eccentric views, paranoid moments, emotional weak spots, overvalued ideas. Who knows, perhaps Terry is right, perhaps his wife and her ex-boyfriend have started up again.

'What were you going to say if you found him?'

'That I knew what he was up to, that he *must* leave her alone.'

'And what would you do if he refused?'

Terry yawns, exposing sharp canines. 'Oh, I hadn't thought about that,' he says unconvincingly.

Suddenly I feel sick of his fencing. We don't have time to try to extract his story now; we have a distressed, violent patient waiting to be seen at the other end of the hospital.

'So have you found him?'

He shakes his head. 'Not yet.' He chuckles mirthlessly. 'I began to think this method wasn't going to work.'

This strange plan about the cars makes me wonder if there is something else going on, some deterioration in the physical stuff of his brain. It's plain to me we need to get him to stay while we dig deeper into the whole story. Letting him out without understanding more does not feel like a safe option, either for him or his wife.

'My wife said she was worried about me, that I should get help.'

'I think she was right, Terry,' I say.

He flinches, as if I have said something hurtful.

'That's when I came up with this plan to scare her.'

'Did you scare her?'

'She didn't tell me his name, if that's what you mean. Just called the ambulance people instead.'

A warm breeze drifts in the window, bringing with it the promise of a summer evening spent outdoors, something I feel we should deny Terry.

'Do you think you need help, Terry?'

Terry blinks and a pained expression flits across his face,

then he recovers and smiles again. 'Need a new wife perhaps?'

'Would you stay for a few hours just so we can have a proper chat?' I ask. 'So that we can find out a bit more about your general health, your background?'

'Of course,' he says. 'Whatever you think best.'

A wicket is taken on the radio; there's a cheer from the crowd, then a shout from the same direction and a muffled thump. The radio is turned off.

'I love her,' Terry says.

We shake hands with him. 'We'll come back in a while.'

'I love her,' he says.

Abdul explains the plan to the ward nurse, Moses. Terry has agreed to a voluntary stay for review by the boss later this afternoon. But he's not to be let out if he asks to leave in the meantime.

At the back of the old-age ward is another heavy door that requires the swipe of an appropriate card. We continue down a short corridor and then another and then suddenly, finally, we have arrived at the 136 Suite.

The 'place of safety' looks a lot like a prison cell. It's about five metres long and three metres wide and contains a single screwed-down bench covered in foam. There are no other furnishings, no ligature points, no decoration. One of the walls is dominated by a huge observation window.

Me, Abdul and the two mental health nurses, Ibrahim and Kimberley, hover in the narrow space on the other side of the polycarbonate window. Together we stare at the large agitated woman with bleach-blonde hair who is pacing around the cell.

'Where have you been?' asks Kimberley. She doesn't sound surprised by our tardiness, more distressed. We shrug. 'This is Caitlin,' she continues, flicking her head to indicate the woman on the other side. 'She's forty-one years old. She has bipolar disorder and seems to be in a manic phase.'

This last clause is made clear as Caitlin runs towards the window, clenched fists raised above her head, and brings them crashing down. The thick polycarb window clatters with her anger. 'Let me out, you fucking cunts. Fucking . . . let me . . . out.' Each word is emphasized by her clattering fists.

Humans are designed to notice if someone in close proximity wants to harm them and it's hard to ignore Caitlin's earth-shattering fury.

'Any psychotic symptoms?' asks Abdul.

'Nothing obvious. She's been agitated like this since she arrived. The computer system's down again so we can't get her old notes at the moment. But we contacted her husband and he's on his way in.'

Kimberley fills us in on the story the police told her when they dropped Caitlin off.

Earlier in the day she was found wandering around the high street swigging from a can of lager and abusing passers-by and someone called the police. She went into a Wetherspoons pub and began screaming at the customers. When the police arrived she got more upset and started shouting and swearing. When they tried to detain her she had punched a policewoman in the face and bitten a policeman's finger down to the bone. Kimberley said he was now in A & E being seen to by the plastic surgeons.

I cautiously glance through the window at the woman.

She is tall and broad, wearing a flimsy vest and skirt in keeping with the sweltering day outside. Her vest has an italicized legend: TIGER GIRL. She is pacing barefoot up and down the length of the cell, muttering to herself. Some bright red high heels stand at one side of the cell. She is sweating heavily. I avert my gaze with the instinctive respect accorded to the violent but too late.

Now Caitlin's form fills the window. Her pale face has glossily painted red lips, the same colour as the shoes. 'What are you looking at, you cunt?'

I can't think of anything helpful to say.

Abdul takes over and speaks through the window. 'Caitlin, we're the psychiatric team. We're here to help you.'

Caitlin sizes him up, then resumes speaking, fists rattling the window to emphasize each syllable. 'Let . . . me . . . out . . .'

'We need to assess your mental state first,' says Abdul.

'I'm gonna kill you,' Caitlin says, and starts smashing at the plastic pane.

We try to resume our professional conversation in front of the pulsating window. The sooner we can assess Caitlin, the sooner we can agree she needs to be sectioned, the sooner we can sedate her, admit her and the sooner we can all get away from her.

After a while Caitlin stops smashing at the window and rests her hands on the glass. I can see long acrylic red nails, four of them snapped in half. Then she resumes her pacing.

Abdul chooses this moment to make his approach. He walks to the door and opens it twenty-five centimetres. He stands with one foot in the cell, one foot outside it. He is on the threshold.

'Caitlin, can I talk to you?' he asks in a calm voice.

'I want a drink.'

'I can get you a drink. And I'd like to talk to you.'

'You're nothing to me. I need a drink and I need to get out. I WANT A DRINK. I WANT TO GET OUT.'

Caitlin moves surprisingly quickly, scooping up a red high-heel shoe in her right hand and launching herself at Abdul from the back of the cell. Abdul moves quickly too. He is back outside and with the door shut before Caitlin brings the shoe heel crashing into it.

Abdul gets on the phone to bring in the consultant. There's no question that Caitlin needs formal assessment for sectioning.

Ibrahim, the nurse, speaks for the first time. He is a large man, calm in demeanour. His pink linen shirt is drenched in sweat. 'We have to get those shoes off her,' he says.

It's true the shoes should have been removed before she was put in the room, but that doesn't seem as important to me now as keeping the door between us closed.

Caitlin has returned to the far side of the cell and resumed her pacing.

Ibrahim moves to the door and opens it with a foot. 'Caitlin,' he says, 'we need those shoes, doll.'

A red shoe comes flying across the room and smashes into the wall above his head. Ibrahim calmly stoops to pick it up. Then Caitlin raises the other shoe above her and runs forward, ready to bring it crashing down on him. Ibrahim dodges smartly back through the door and the shoe comes hurtling down on the other side.

The sliding door to the 136 Suite opens and another nurse ushers in a large man wearing a long football shirt, a pair of khaki shorts and green flip-flops.

'I'm Caitlin's husband, Aaron,' he says.

We all shake hands.

'I'm so glad you've got her. I've been looking for her all day.'

He listens patiently while we relay the story of Caitlin's morning.

'We're having trouble getting her to engage with us,' says Abdul.

'I'm sorry about this,' Aaron says, rubbing his brow. 'It happens whenever the anniversary comes. I tried to warn them.'

'Have a seat,' I say, waving him towards a chair.

'It's fine. I'd rather stand.'

'Some water?' asks Ibrahim.

Caitlin's husband takes the plastic beaker absently and drains it.

'Which anniversary?' I ask.

'Caitlin had a daughter. She drowned in the bath when she was three while a friend was supposed to be looking after her. Caitlin's never forgiven herself.'

I look over at Caitlin, muttering to herself in the corner of the cell.

'Usually her bipolar is well controlled,' says her husband, 'but whenever the anniversary approaches she stops sleeping, gets agitated and it becomes impossible to get her to take the medication. It's as if reality becomes too much to bear. I told her doctor we needed to admit her. It happens every year. But he said there isn't the capacity to get people in until things get worse . . . The funny thing is, she thinks she's on top of the world when she's like this. It's amazing the tricks the mind can play. I tried to stay with her but my work said I had to come in or I'd get sacked. We can't afford that. So I left her and crossed my fingers . . .'

We open the cell door and Aaron goes inside.

'Hi, Caitlin,' he says. 'I've found you.'

'Aaron,' Caitlin almost shouts, relieved. 'How'd you find me?'

'They called me.' He gestures towards us, all trying to look inconspicuous behind the large window. 'They're trying to help you. You need help, Caitlin.'

She stands still. Tears trickle from her eyes and mix with the sweat on her cheeks.

'How are you doing, Caitlin?' Aaron says, and closes the distance between them and hugs her. 'Come and sit with me,' he says.

She wanders over, meek as a lamb, and they sit on the padded bench together.

'Hey, don't worry,' Aaron says, holding her tight. 'Don't worry.'

The consultant comes into the suite from the outside entrance expecting mayhem. We point at the calm scene in the cell.

'Her husband,' I say.

The consultant nods her head. 'Well done, guys.'

Abdul stays to write his notes. I leave the way I have come. Threading through the wards and corridors of the mental hospital, taking several wrong turnings then reorienting myself. Through the old-age ward, the male ward, the female ward, out past the intensive care section. Through and past all the suffering.

I'm almost back at the security desk when a woman in the corridor stops me. She is middle-aged and dressed in the kind of smart shoulder-padded suit that I thought had died out with Margaret Thatcher. She looks lost.

'Can I help you?' I ask.

'Yes please,' she says. 'I'm looking for my husband. He was brought in a few hours ago; his name is Terry—'

'Oh, you're Terry's wife?' I say and introduce myself.

'How is he?' she asks.

'He's safe,' I say neutrally. 'We want to understand him better. It'll be useful to hear what you can tell us.'

'He's always been very private,' she says. 'I don't really understand him myself.'

'It's easy to get lost in this place,' I say, and explain in the simplest terms how to get there.

I walk on, thinking about Caitlin and Terry. Both haunted by ghosts from the past. One only able to be comforted by her partner, the other only able to be tormented by his.

I recover my bag from security and head out of the main entrance and on to the front steps. I stop, blinded and dazed by the bright sunlight. My eyes adjust to the outside world. Behind me the most extreme mental disquiet of the city is packed into a chaotically assembled set of boxes. The roots and tendrils of this suffering are woven through the city around me.

At my approach the cat with the three white socks stretches on its windowsill and stands up. Then we both head off into the sultry summer evening.

Octopus Trap

Helena was dragged out of the river that runs through the meadows by passers-by. It was about ten on a warm midsummer evening but she was fully clothed and they thought she was drowning. When they got her to the riverbank she was agitated and by the time the paramedics arrived she was screaming so loudly that the horses in the meadows were spooked and started galloping away.

At the hospital it is clear that she is high on something. Her pupils are big black coins, her heart rate is galloping, she has a fever, and her limbs posture stiffly. She is so agitated the security team have to hold her down so we can get the cannula in. We give her a shot of something to calm her down, send off bloods, then leave her in a cubicle to sleep.

When I shout for Alex, the next patient, three times over the humming crowd, no one answers. I place his triage card back on the pile but one of the nurses working nearby points and says, 'He's that one in the Stone Roses T-shirt.'

I wave and a stocky fellow stands up with buzz-cut hair, shorts and a T-shirt all green and white Jackson Pollock paint splashes punctuated with three slices of lemon.

'I'm sorry,' I say. 'I called.'

The man smiles at me. 'I'm deaf,' he says in a slightly mushy voice. 'I must have missed your lips moving.'

Sitting opposite me in the cubicle, Alex describes excruciating stomach pains that came on suddenly earlier today and have persisted into the night. The rest of the history he gives is nondescript and provides no clues as to what might be going on.

'I've never felt anything like it before,' he says, pulling up the T-shirt and putting his hands behind his head as he lies on the couch. 'It lasted all day.'

As I press into his tummy it seems reassuringly soft.

'I love the Stone Roses,' I say, and to my surprise at this Alex starts sobbing, tears pouring out of his eyes, nose streaming, body shaking with emotion.

I grab a block of tissues from the sink dispenser and get him sitting upright and hand them to him. 'What's going on?' I ask as he dabs at his face.

'I'm sorry,' he says. 'The Roses were my girlfriend's favourite band . . .'

'What happened?'

'She broke up with me.'

'When did this happen?'

'Today,' he says.

'I'm so sorry,' I say.

Together we work out that the stomach pains started immediately after she made it clear that she wasn't going to change her mind. Alex was so strung out he hadn't made the connection. We talk about what he should do, who he can talk to, how to get through this time. Just talking about her seems to make him feel better. And, after a while, he smiles through the tears, and says, 'The pain's gone.'

*

The next patient, Dorothy, is already in a cubicle, lying on the bed, thin, frail and grey, looking straight ahead. Her impassive face looks almost like a mask.

'How are you feeling, Dorothy?'

She lies there staring straight ahead not seeming to have heard. I can see from her triage card that she has Parkinson's Disease, which tends to slow everything down: movement, speech, facial expression. I wait patiently and I can just see her lips begin to move when her husband, sitting next to her, interjects.

'She's not been able to get out of bed for the last two days,' he says.

Dorothy's face settles back to its previously impassive state.

'How are *you* feeling, Dorothy?' I ask again.

'I think she's getting a bit of a cough,' her husband pipes up. 'She gets chest infections easily, you see.'

'Dorothy, how's your breathing?'

'Oh, her breathing's fine,' her husband says.

'Do you mind letting Dorothy answer?'

'No, of course,' he says. 'It's just it's difficult for her to talk. She likes me to talk for her. I'm Jim, by the way.' He holds out his hand and I shake it.

Despite this Jim cannot restrain himself from answering my next three questions before Dorothy gets a chance. Frustrated, I lean in towards her and say, 'I just want to hear how you're feeling.'

This time Jim restrains himself. We watch Dorothy as in slow motion she makes the gargantuan effort to respond. Eventually her mouth starts moving and her voice comes, quiet and slow, each syllable carefully enunciated and slightly slurred.

'Just . . . tired,' she finally says, and then there's another long pause. 'Nothing . . . else.'

'Do you mind if I talk to your husband about your condition, Dorothy?'

'She won't mind,' Jim says benevolently. 'Her condition makes it hard for her to speak.'

I smile at him and wait doggedly for her to answer. There's another long pause.

'No . . . that's . . . fine.'

Jim smiles with satisfaction. 'You see.'

I ask her husband about the home situation. He does everything for her. Prepares her food, washes her, takes her to the toilet, gets her in and out of the car, drives her to bingo.

'We don't have any carers,' he says. 'She doesn't want strangers around. But I'm happy to do it all. We've been married forty-five years. We watch snooker and Formula One together; she likes whatever's on,' he says. Tears well in his eyes. 'I'd do anything for her,' he says.

Contemplating the enormity of day-to-day life for Dorothy and Jim I feel tears pricking my own eyes.

Examining her I get a sense of just how weak she really is. Through underuse there is little muscle left. When not moving, her limbs are tremulous, rigid. When moving, everything is sluggish, delayed. All this is consistent with her Parkinson's. But the examination doesn't produce any clear explanation for why she's recently slowed down so much. *Sometimes these deteriorations just happen in Parkinson's,* I think to myself, and we probably need to tweak the medications and get her reviewed later at home.

Dorothy's eyes bulge out at me. It must be so frustrating to be stuck here, trapped inside this body, this situation, unable to look after yourself, even speak for yourself, let alone gain the joy of caring for others. Thank goodness she has this devoted husband helping her at every step of the way.

'We should get a urine sample and a chest X-ray,' I say, 'and if those and the blood tests are normal the best plan would be to get you ho–'

Suddenly I hear shouting through the curtain. I rush out to see the patient from the river running across the department, screaming. Two burly black-clad security guards are chasing after her. Eventually one of them pins her down.

'Helena,' I say when I catch up, 'don't worry, we're here to look after you.'

'Let me go,' she screams. 'Let me go.'

'We can't do that,' I say. 'We're keeping you here for your own safety. Why don't we get you back to the bed and we can give you something to calm you down?'

Helena doesn't seem to be listening, her eyes aren't focused on us; she looks like a wild animal, as if she is being hunted.

'Where am I?' she screams, scratching and kicking out at the security men. 'Who are you?'

'You're at the — Hospital,' I say as calmly as I can. 'We're looking after you; you just need to sleep.'

One of the security men pins Helena down on the floor, still shouting and sobbing. We erect a temporary barrier of wheeled screens round her to shield her from the eyes of the waiting room. Eventually she tires and weakens and the security team carry her back to her bed-space where we draw up some medicine and give her another shot. Soon she is sleeping again.

*

Before I can get back to Dorothy I am asked to assess a patient suffering from chest pain.

Frieda is an overweight middle-aged white woman with no previous medical problems. She is sweating and looking frightened.

'The pain came on this afternoon, when I was in the garden,' she says. 'It started gradually but now it feels like an elephant's sitting on my chest.'

'Were you walking around when the pain came on?' I ask.

'No, just sitting reading a book,' she says.

The electronic heart trace that was done as soon as she arrived looks normal, but a rapid turnaround blood test suggests her heart muscle is damaged and leaking protein. I get a repeat of the heart trace and this time some of the waves suggest that electricity is not moving through her heart in the uniform way it should. I bleep the cardiologists and ask them to take her urgently to the cath lab to look at the state of the arteries that feed blood to the heart.

I explain to Frieda what they will do there, and that there is probably a blockage in an artery that needs to be cleared. I ask if there is anyone we can call to be with her and tears well up in her eyes and she shakes her head.

'My husband died,' she says.

'I'm so sorry,' I say. 'When did that happen?'

'Two days ago,' she says. 'We're burying him Saturday.'

The porters arrive to whip her off to the cath lab.

'You're going to be fine,' I say. 'They'll look after you.'

Dorothy's tests all look normal and when I come back to her she is lying rigid in bed, her mask-like face staring straight ahead and her husband is nowhere to be seen. Alone in the anonymous hospital cubicle she looks even more vulnerable. I explain that I can't find a reason for her deterioration but the best thing would be for her to go home and be seen by the Parkinson's nurse the next day.

'Is that OK?' I ask, and wait for what feels like an age with the busy department humming behind me.

There is no reply.

'How are you feeling?' I ask her, and wait as, eyes bulging, Dorothy marshals her damaged nervous system into producing a response. Finally her lips start to move and the words come out in a whisper. 'He . . . bullies me.'

I feel shocked. What have I stumbled across here? And how can we possibly untangle it? Carers get exhausted, snappy with their charges; the cared for get sick of being cared for. The frustration for everyone is immense. And, of course, people do just sometimes bully others, vulnerable people especially. Then there's the fact that Parkinson's can sometimes affect the emotions and the mind. And what really is the alternative to her husband Jim looking after her?

'I'm sorry to hear that,' I say.

Someone who doesn't have a waiting room full of people behind them needs to take time and listen to Dorothy.

'Would it be helpful if we get you to a ward overnight so you can talk to someone about this in the morning?'

I watch her face carefully and after what feels an age she nods.

By five in the morning we've dug our way through most of the waiting room. The nurse comes to tell me that Helena has woken up again. This time she is calmer. The fever has gone and her heart rate has settled. Her pupils are still large and she still looks haunted.

'How are you feeling?' I ask, perched on the end of the bed.

She turns away from me and pulls the blanket tightly round her.

'If you can tell me what you took last night, it would be helpful,' I say.

She is silent. I am exhausted, so I just sit there, listening to the beeps of the machines and the breathing of the sleeping humans around us.

'The dealer said it was MDMA.' Her voice comes from the bed. 'I didn't care what it was. I would have taken anything.'

'Thank you,' I say, and absorb this piece of information, which fits with all the symptoms we saw. Given how she looks now things should continue to improve.

'Why did you go into the river?'

'I don't know,' she says, and shivers. 'I remember I was talking to one of the horses, stroking its cheek, when all of a sudden it bolted and I suddenly felt crazy . . .'

'You weren't trying to kill yourself?'

She is still facing away. I stay sitting there. 'I don't remember,' she says.

'How are you feeling now?'

There's another long pause.

'Sad,' she says.

'What's making you sad?' I ask.

She lies there, clenched in on herself under the sheet, still resolutely facing away under the dimmed strip lights. 'She left me,' she says.

'I'm sorry,' I say.

'I didn't think she would just leave me.'

'Do you want to talk about it?' I ask.

Still facing away she shakes her head.

I go to get Helena a cup of tea and see a tired-looking cardiologist in purple scrubs wandering into the department wheeling a large ultrasound machine behind her like a mechanical pet.

'You were the doctor who sent us Frieda, weren't you?' she says.

'The woman with chest pain,' I say. 'How is she?'

'Fine. But I wanted to show you something we don't see every day,' she says. 'We took her to the cath lab. Her coronary arteries were as clean as a whistle. But this is what the echo showed.'

She presses a few buttons and plays a recorded clip on the screen of the machine that shows the beating of Frieda's heart, rhythmically pulsating in black and white.

Usually the largest of the four chambers, the left ventricle, squeezes in an organized fashion that begins at the top and spreads evenly down to the tip from where blood is forced around the body, all the way up around the brain, all the way down to the toes. In Frieda's left ventricle the contraction starts from the top as normal but the lower half has ballooned out and stubbornly refuses to contract. This explains her low blood pressure and the chest pain, the blood test and ECG results.

'That's takotsubo,' says the cardiologist, pausing the image so the ballooning tip of the heart is freeze-framed and tracing its outline with her finger. 'It's the Japanese word for an octopus trap. The doctor who first described it thought the heart looked like the pots fishermen place on the seabed to catch octopus.'

She clicks a button and I watch as Frieda's heart starts beating again on the screen, the rhythmic pulsing, the unexpected stop. The large section of her heart is quivering, on strike, an octopus trap.

'It usually happens after a stressful experience,' the cardiologist says. 'We think the sudden release of adrenaline stuns that bit of the heart.'

'Her husband,' I say.

'Frieda told us he died. That'd do it.'

'You know when you get those shifts where almost all the patients seem to have the same problem?' I say. 'One way or the other mine has been dominated by heartbreak.'

'It's been a while since I did anything but hearts,' the cardiologist says and smiles.

'Is Frieda going to make it?'

'Oh yes, she'll recover,' the cardiologist says, taking the brake off the machine in anticipation of her next case, 'but it'll take time.'

Prison

The dark brick entrance to the Victorian prison is fringed with green and red tinsel to mark long-past festivities. The security guard has an angry red rash festooned round his neck, and after a cursory search he lets me and Denise, the prison doctor, in.

Denise is a short, blonde-haired woman with a serious cast to her lined face. She leads me inside.

Because of the low winter sun and the three-metre-high, one-metre-thick walls most of the site is in shade, and layers of ice coat the ground where outside there was none.

There is not a soul to be seen as we amble, bone-achingly cold, through the many perimeter zones. The prison is laid out with concentrically spaced buildings and walls nestling within each other like Russian dolls. Each low-slung building block and high perimeter fence we pass through acts as a new barrier from the outside world and freedom. Between each zone a solid metal gate clanks shut and the prison doctor turns with her jangling bunch of keys to lock them behind us as if carefully whittling out a cancerous mass. In the peripheral zones we can still hear the birds twittering high in the trees outside where the winter sun falls, but as we get further inside the trees become more distant and the birds fall silent.

We enter the remand wing that houses the prisoners who have been arrested but are still awaiting trial. Some of them have already been waiting in prison for months, Denise tells me, some over a year. We pass through a couple of magnetically secured reinforced plastic doors that bear the scratches and cracks of previous assaults and suddenly the place is warm and bright and loud with shouted insults, greetings, complaints and the crashing of cell doors.

Standing in the vestibule of the remand wing we are five locked doors from freedom and in front of us is another large door, this one comprised of thick vertical bars leading into the remand cell block where prisoners are queuing to get their breakfast. The hot fug of the central heating, the bodies, the oven trays of bacon, the banter wafts through the bars.

'Same old swill.'

'Look like you been catching a ride, Tony.'

'Shut your mouth.'

'Watch out for the rub-down.'

Next to the barred door is an office with a laminated counter facing us in the vestibule and on the other side a small hatch giving on to the cell block at which stands a slender whey-faced man with a stubbly head. Someone in the office brings a small plastic beaker containing a pill in it and puts it down on the hatch. The prisoner tosses the pill into his mouth, takes a sip of water and swallows theatrically. Then he opens his mouth wide to prove to the attendant that he has swallowed it and that the carefully crafted chemicals will enter the bloodstream of their intended recipient.

'They still sometimes vomit them back up and sell them,' Denise mumbles to me, 'but it lowers the value.'

She leads me into a small corridor off the vestibule and

introduces me to Orla, a tall, skinny serious-looking woman with no make-up and a pair of wire-framed spectacles. Orla is from Belfast. She has been working as a nurse on the drugs, rehab and prison beats of medicine for thirty years in Northern Ireland and England.

'We're processing the new remand prisoners,' Denise explains. 'They've been arrested within the last twenty-four hours so they're new to the prison. Orla takes down their details and their recreational drug and medication use on the outside. Then any vital prescriptions or drug replacements we carry on in here. Basically Orla does all the hard work, then I prescribe.'

Denise walks off to her room next door to do some paper-work and I follow Orla into a narrow sliver of a room. We sit at the desk that is nearer the door to give us a better chance of escape if the prisoners kick off.

At the far end of the room is a low-slung chair in which is folded a tall man.

After Orla has identified the man from his notes he speaks.

'I shouldn't be here,' he volunteers calmly. 'They got the wrong guy.'

He is of indeterminate middle age, a gaunt face with coffee-coloured skin smooth like putty applied to the skull beneath. He speaks slowly and surely in a deep, rasping voice. 'I was defending myself.'

The man looks professorial, his lazy eyes blinking behind wire-rimmed specs with dark lenses. The professor is lying right back in the low prison chair, his legs stretching out towards us, arms casually hanging at his side. He looks like he's sizing us up. He is still and calm, and haloed by the rays of weak winter sun emanating through the window behind, so that he looks like some sort of holy praying mantis.

'We aren't here to talk about that,' says Orla in a broad Northern Irish accent.

'I'll talk about what I want to talk about,' he says mildly.

'Then we'll have to stop right here,' she says, 'and pick it up tomorrow.'

He looks us over and slowly licks his upper lip. 'Well, that's a shame,' he says, a darker tone entering his voice. And then just like that he smiles. 'Let's try your way,' he says, 'and see where we get.'

'Good idea,' Orla says.

'Yessss,' he says, a purr of dissatisfaction.

'We just want to discuss your medical history,' says Orla, scarcely masking her distaste at his desire to dwell on the crime he says he didn't commit.

He ignores her and starts calmly explaining the large quantities of illegal drugs he has been using outside. 'I was using dark,' he says, 'light, K, X, Candy, you name it.'

'How much heroin?' Orla asks.

'Ohhh, about five hundred quids' worth a week. The crack about the same. Light to go up, dark to come down.'

I can't stop myself from doing the sums in my head. Fifty grand a year? That habit would need a very well-paid job or a lot of theft and robbery to bankroll it.

The professor looks at us appraisingly. 'Oh, and I smoke.'

'That's bad for your health,' Orla says. 'We can help you quit if you'd like.'

'Which?' he says.

'The smoking.'

'And the rest, miss?' he asks ironically.

'The rest you *will* be quitting,' Orla says.

'Really?' the professor says. 'You seem reasonable, miss, and intelligent, so you know that'd be dangerous.'

'How do you mean?' Orla asks.

'I'm coming down; my bones are aching, miss.'

'Really?'

'Yes,' he says, clutching at his body with his long arms. 'I feel sick. I'm clucking.'

'No, you're not,' she says sharply.

His face contorts with anger. 'How dare you tell me what I'm feeling?' he shouts. He's trembling with rage and leaning forward in his chair, looking as if he might leap up at any moment. 'You can't jump into my body and know what I'm feeling,' the professor rages.

'I'm just saying that your urine tests show no trace of opiates, no trace of coke derivatives, no trace of benzodiazepines,' Orla says calmly.

'The tests must be wrong,' the professor shouts, still trembling. And then as quickly as the anger comes it subsides, and the professor folds himself back into the chair, and he rubs a lightly stubbled cheek with his hand.

'Don't tell me what I'm feeling,' he growls again. 'I'm telling you, miss. I'm cluckin' and I need methadone.'

Orla looks at him over the wire rims of her spectacles. 'The tests are accurate. Now what about your medical history?'

The professor sets to shaking his head and muttering, then recovers his poise. 'I've been diagnosed with dangerous and severe personality disorder,' he says, looking through the smoked lenses of his specs. 'Do you know what that means?'

Orla doesn't say anything.

'It means I'm a very dangerous character,' he says, 'and don't care who gets hurt.'

'Is that right?' Orla says.

'Yes, miss, that's right,' he says, becoming rigid once more. 'Are you trying to rile me?'

'No,' says Orla, 'but I hear this kind of thing quite a lot.'

'Do you?'

'And I'd rather just get your medical history without the commentary,' she says.

I'm impressed by Orla's coolness in front of this intimidating character, but part of me wishes she wouldn't be so confrontational.

'OK,' he says, 'I'm prescribed codeine and pregabalin by my GP for shoulder pain. And I'm on mirtazapine for anxiety and depression.' He chuckles mirthlessly. 'Life can get depressing when you have dangerous and severe personality disorder.'

'Which pharmacy provides you that?'

He gives the address of a pharmacy in a distant town, then Orla picks up the phone and dials their number.

He sounds perfectly plausible, I think. And he must know he'll get found out if he's lying, so why would he bother?

Orla chats to the pharmacist then rings off. 'They've never heard of you,' she says.

He shakes his head. 'They must have made a mistake. I'm sofa-surfing at the moment so I move around a lot.'

Orla purses her lips. 'I don't think so.'

'So,' says the professor, voice laden with menace, 'I'm cluckin', I'm in agony with my damaged shoulder and are you telling me that you're not going to give me any drugs while I'm here?'

'The doctor might want to prescribe you some ibuprofen,' Orla says.

'Ibuprofen?' he flares up. 'Ibuprofen? You're a character, miss. You're antagonistic, miss. You got a problem with men, miss? I think you do.'

'Please don't disrespect me,' Orla says. 'I'm trying to help you. We try to get people off drugs in here, not put people on them.'

'You ever done any time?' the man sneers.

'No,' she says.

'I don't think you'd last long,' he says, 'with the attitude you've got. Time is long in here, miss.'

'I'm sure it is,' Orla says, 'but if you're clean when you get out, you've got a better chance of getting life back on track.'

Some rays of sun penetrate the window and cast the professor in shadow. His eyes glint through the smoky spectacles. 'Who says my life is off track?' he says.

Orla shrugs.

'Do you know why I'm here?' he asks.

'No,' Orla says. 'I really don't need to either.'

'GBH,' the professor says. 'She's in hospital in a bad way.' He fixes his gaze on Orla. 'Nothing to do with me, of course.'

'Well, that's that,' Orla says. 'If you wait outside to see the doctor, she'll come to you soon.'

The professor unfolds himself from the chair and stands, towering over us as he slowly files past in the narrow room. Menace on his face, crackling with anger.

To my disappointment rather than being escorted away by a guard he just goes and sits on a bench in the corridor directly behind the door of our room.

Orla turns to me and raises an ironic eyebrow, as if to say

'what did you think about that?', then turns to fill out her notes.

I ponder the professor and what I've just seen. The sense I got from him was that he genuinely couldn't care less about either of us. There are no grudges, no guilt, no hard or soft feelings either way, he does just enough of what is in his limited range of tricks to try to get what he wants. We are nothing to him and it's hard to find empathy for people like that.

The next two patients' stories follow much the same script. Carefully delineating the vast quantities of illegal drugs they've apparently been taking when outside and the medical drugs they are apparently prescribed for depression and pain, always from the same small group of meds that are known to give a buzz or a high. Each time they make the claims with a high degree of conviction, though neither of them are as plausible or as menacing as the professor. Each time the urine tests have no trace of these substances, and the pharmacy where they tell us they get their meds has no record of them. This is all part of some strange standard operating procedure, I begin to realize. When the second prisoner is confronted with the facts he just folds immediately, smiles, shrugs and leaves. The third prisoner rants and raves, swears that the urine tests and the pharmacy computers are faulty, but not with as much conviction as the professor. He walks out and sits outside on a bench with the other two. Through the thick glass I can see them swearing angrily to each other and gesticulating towards our room.

'Shouldn't we have a guard out there with the prisoners?' I ask Orla.

'We should,' she says, 'but as usual we don't. The whole place is chronically understaffed. The guard only comes when they're free.' She seems unbothered. 'Did you notice a pattern?' she asks me.

'Yes,' I say, 'it was exactly the same for each one.'

She nods her head. 'A lot of them try it on and I know it's dull for them. But it won't help them later on if they get an opiate habit in here.'

'But are the urine tests any good?' I ask.

'They're the ones we always use,' Orla says. 'And, you heard them, they were lying about the prescription drugs, the street drugs. They'd say anything.'

She looks at me defensively. Perhaps she's detected something in my tone. It must be so frustrating having these prisoners lying and acting out constantly. But still there was something weirdly confrontational about the whole business.

'This is all a bit repetitive for you,' she says. 'If you'd like you could sit in with Denise for a while.'

'That'd be great,' I say.

'She's just on the left out there, the next door along.'

'Sure,' I say.

She hands me the notes she's made on the first three prisoners. And I thank her for letting me sit with her.

I open the door and nod to the prisoners on the bench, who go silent as I emerge. I knock on the door to the left. Nothing happens. I try the handle but the door's locked. Peering through the oblong window I can see Denise behind a desk on the phone and she holds up a finger as if to say 'one minute'. So I sit on a chair in the corridor a few metres away from the prisoners on the bench. They stare at me sullenly.

'Bitch wouldn't give me anything,' I can just hear the third prisoner whispering to the others.

'Yep,' says prisoner two.

I try to ignore them.

I do wonder about these drugs tests. It's true, as Orla says, that the men seemed to be lying, but it doesn't mean nothing they said was true. Most drugs tests are designed to catch people who are abusing drugs, and the sensitivity threshold is set high so the tests don't catch people unfairly. For that reason they may not be very good at ruling drug use out.

I hear the professor whispering off to my left. 'Said I wasn't cluckin'. As if the damn bitch knows what I'm feeling.'

'Yeah,' says the second prisoner, 'she doesn't give a shit.'

'I'm in for GBH,' the professor mutters. 'She's proper fucked up,' he says. 'I didn't do it; they've got nothing on me, but I'm gonna be here for a while.'

The second prisoner chuckles bitterly at the unknown woman's fate. 'I'm fucked, mate,' he says. 'I broke my parole again. I'm comin' in for a long time.'

'Me too,' says the third prisoner. Then he whispers something and the others chuckle.

'Yeah. If they're not going to give us anything –' The second prisoner's voice goes quieter, and I think I hear him say, 'We should take it.'

I feel the adrenaline scooting through me. The professor starts whispering again. I am hyper-aware of these men sitting between me and freedom. My paranoia tells me the professor is either plotting or provoking the other prisoners to harm me, Denise and Orla.

'I've got nothing to lose, mate,' I hear the second prisoner say, a little louder. Do they think I can't hear them? Are they doing all this just to wind me up, or do they just not care that I can hear?

To my relief the door to Denise's room opens and she beckons me in. This room is a bit larger, and it's a relief to have more space and have the door closed behind us, though I'm conscious that the prisoners still block our exit. Denise takes the paperwork Orla has written from me and starts reading it over the top of specs pushed to the tip of her nose. She looks exhausted, her face pale and lined.

'Did you find that interesting?' she asks.

'I wasn't expecting to hear so many confessions of drug abuse,' I say.

'Oh, that,' she says. 'The days must drag in here. They either want it for themselves, or to barter for other things.'

'Are the drugs tests sensitive?' I ask.

She ponders the question then shrugs. 'I'm not actually sure.'

'Orla's pretty tough,' I say.

'Yes.' Denise chuckles and shakes her head. 'She's determined to help them get clean. The problem is we don't have proper resources for rehab and the place is awash in recreational drugs. The main difference it makes is that the ones we prescribe will add to the pool.'

'And they're all after antidepressants and neuropathic painkillers,' I say.

'Those are the prescription drugs that have a reputation for giving a buzz, so they have a value in here too, and I've no doubt that's why they're asking for them, along with the opiates and the benzos.' She suppresses a yawn. 'But the truth is, given their backgrounds, their lifestyles, most of them are probably depressed and quite possibly in pain, but have never been to the doctor about it and are just self-medicating in the outside world.'

'So they're actually after things they might need although that's not why they want them,' I say.

'In a lot of cases, yes,' Denise says.

She starts flicking through Orla's notes. And I finally say the thing that's been bothering me.

'The prisoners outside seem quite on edge.'

Denise looks up, consternation across her face. 'I don't like the way they leave them free in these areas,' she says. 'What do you mean?'

I describe what I think I've heard. 'I don't know if I'm being paranoid,' I add.

Denise seems unhappy at the news. 'Let's get things moving,' she says.

She jumps up and walks round the desk, keys clanking at her belt, opens the door and beckons.

The professor ambles in watchfully, like a cat, muscles tensed and Denise hurriedly closes the door behind him, hovering for a moment at the window to look out at the other two prisoners who remain on the bench between us and the first of five doors that lead to our freedom.

The professor stands looming in the middle of the room, strangely still. He seems about to speak, to initiate something, but Denise gets in first.

'So, I can see from my colleague's notes that you have a bad shoulder and anxiety,' she says.

'Yeah,' says the professor gruffly.

'How did you hurt it?'

'Oh, some bloke jumped me five years ago. I didn't have a

chance,' he croons. 'He damaged the nerves; it's been painful ever since.'

'And we can't find the prescription at the pharmacy,' Denise says.

'Some mistake,' the professor says huskily. 'Some balls-up.'

'That can sometimes happen,' Denise says. 'Now let's have a look at this shoulder.'

A communication seems to have taken place and the professor seems more relaxed now. Automatically he seems to stiffen up on his left side. Denise examines his shoulder and almost every movement he makes provokes grimaces of significant pain.

'We need to try to get you some physiotherapy . . .' Denise says, then she pauses. There is tension in the air. 'But that'll take some time to arrange. And while we're waiting we need to help with the pain. I don't think we need the codeine, but gabapentin is probably a good idea.'

The professor tilts his head on one side as if considering a proposition, and after a few seconds he nods his head. 'And what about the mirtazapine for my anxiety?' he asks. 'Pharmacy didn't know about that either.'

'Gabapentin is good for anxiety as well if we get the dose right,' Denise says.

The professor looks around the room cautiously then back at Denise. Then, as if he's decided he's not going to get anything else, he relaxes. 'I think you need to talk to that . . . to miss next door about her attitude.' He snorts with triumph, eyes glinting behind the smoked glasses.

'She was doing her job,' Denise says.

She looks worn out, her shoulders hunched, as she scribbles the prescription that will go to the room next door, which will summon the professor three times a day to the hatch to be given the pills and water and to be watched as he swallows them for the buzz or conceals and barters them in exchange for something else. Things to help while away the days, weeks, months or years inside.

'And,' she mutters almost to herself, 'I think I'm doing mine.'

Arrhythmia

Rebecca and I head to Cardiology Ward A to find two men with damaged hearts.

Alastair and Steve are lying on either side of a two-person bay, each propped up on pillows in bed, each wearing a thin violet hospital gown, each attached to a cardiac monitor. The soles of their feet, covered in green blankets, face each other across the ward corridor. A cursory glance at the monitors shows that while Alastair's heart is beating at regular tempo and rhythm Steve's is cantering along too fast.

They both look well enough, and they're talking to each other across the gap about the best openings to a Rolling Stones song.

'"Under My Thumb",' Alastair says in a clipped voice that speaks of tennis, expensive schools and high-level meetings. He is sitting propped up on his pillows; he looks about sixty years old, with a tanned face, fine wrinkles, wavy brown hair and gold-rimmed specs on the end of his nose. 'That drum riff at the start just plunges you straight in . . .' He uses his index fingers as beaters and taps out a drumbeat on the pink newspaper resting on his lap.

'Can't agree, mate,' Steve says from the opposite bed in a London growl, redolent of football, graft and fist fights. Steve is an ox of a man with sallow Caucasian skin, stubble on his head, a four-inch scar across one temple and a roaring blue lion inked on one muscly forearm. A red-top newspaper is folded on the bedside table.

'"Can't You Hear Me Knockin'"', that's the most bluesy openin' of any song, full stop.'

Steve picks up an imaginary guitar and starts rhythmically strumming it, and nodding his head in time to the silent beat.

Alastair picks up his gold fountain pen and glasses case and starts tapping them away on his pink newspaper in time with Steve.

'Which one shall I go for?' whispers Rebecca.

'Take your pick,' I say. 'Leave me whoever.'

'I'm sorry to interrupt,' Rebecca says, smiling and walking up to Steve's bed.

'Scuse me, Ally,' Steve lobs across the bay, 'important business, but I'll be back for the B-side,' and he chuckles.

'Ally's a good guy,' he says to us, 'likes the Stones . . .' Here he lowers his voice to a stage whisper, making sure his bandmate can still hear. 'Not a clue about music really.'

Alastair grins from behind his newspaper.

Rebecca's in the lead for this one. 'We're medical students and were wondering if you'd mind talking to us.'

'Course,' Steve says in a jovial tone, shuffling his bulk back and sitting up straighter. 'Watcha wanna know?'

Rebecca asks him why he's in hospital.

'I died last night,' he says eyes open wide. 'My heart stopped.'

Rebecca tries to conceal her surprise. 'A cardiac arrest?' she says. 'Do you know why it happened?'

Steve yawns and reveals rows of strong nicotine-yellow

teeth, then looks sheepish. 'My fault,' he says. 'I took something.'

'What?' Rebecca asks.

'Stuff called VanillaSky. I bought it off Wayne, my mate, a sachet of white powder. I'd never had it before and I didn't really know how much to take . . . Pretty fuckin' stupid, I know, pardon my French . . . But I guess a lot of my life's been like that . . .' And at that Steve seems to drift off into his own thoughts.

We can hear the soft beep of the cardiac monitors, the smell of the lunchtime mashed potato and gravy drifts through the ward, and out of the window a large river pours water down towards the sea. I look at Steve's eyes; his pupils are tiny, dwarfed by pale blue irises, much smaller than you'd expect given the gloom of the room. The effect of the drugs is still playing out in his system.

'What happened?' Rebecca prompts.

'Oh, sorry,' he says. 'Just thinking. What 'appened? Well, we were under the flyover, getting comfy on the cider, arguin' about the football, then I took some of this VanillaSky – stupid fucking name. Wayne said for a good long buzz to wrap it in a cigarette paper and eat it so I did, and after half an hour it didn't seem to be doing anything so I ate some more and snorted some. It still didn't seem to be doing anything and I was about to finish it off when I began burnin' up, and feeling out of it.'

He rubs a hand vigorously on his stubbly scalp. 'Then I got confused. I didn't know where the hell I was. At one point I thought my mate Wayne was trying to kill me so I tried to attack him, then my heart started racing, and my chest began hurting. That's the last thing I remember until I woke up here in A & E.'

'Wow,' Rebecca says.

'Apparently I collapsed to the ground,' Steve continues in a matter-of-fact way. 'Dead, basically. My mate called the ambulance and started bouncin' up and down on me chest. Still bloody hurts,' he says, poking at his ribs through the thin lilac hospital gown with thick fingers. 'Luckily for me they were quick and did their thing with the old electricity and brought me back,' he says. 'I got a shock. I don't like hospitals.' And then anxiously he adds, 'No offence.'

'None taken,' Rebecca says, smiling.

'I'm waiting for tests on the heart today.'

'And how are you feeling now?' asks Rebecca.

'I feel fine,' he says, running a coarse hand over his stubbly head. 'Embarrassed. Lucky.'

Rebecca stands there, thinking. I like the way she is happy to be silent with the patients to acknowledge the gravity of their situation rather than rushing on and away from it. I can tell she is deciding which direction to move the conversation.

'Why did you take the drug?' she asks eventually.

'To pass the time,' he says. 'When you're on the street you'll take anything.' He shakes his head. 'Though I ain't taking that one again.'

'That sounds sensible,' Rebecca says. 'How long have you been on the street?'

'On and off about a year,' he says. 'To be honest it's getting me down. I've got to clean myself up and get a place.'

Rebecca pauses again. 'What's stopping you?'

He pauses for a moment and stares into the distance, retreating into his mind, and when he speaks he is less animated and he sounds exhausted. 'Lots of things.'

'Why did you end up on the street?'

Steve turns and fixes Rebecca intently with his eyes, large cornflower irises and pinpoint pupils, before he answers. He seems interested in her reaction.

'Lots of reasons. It's strange where life takes you. I was in the army,' he says, and names a particular regiment then gives a rude nickname for it. And then, as if to pre-empt a question, 'I'm done with all that. I got a medical discharge . . .' He looks away.

We stand in silence again. It seems like he doesn't want to talk about it any more. Rebecca decides to switch the line of enquiry, so she begins asking about his previous health, family health problems, some social stuff, then she asks if she can examine him.

I watch as she takes his hand between hers and stares intently at different aspects of it. He has two nicotine-stained fingers; his fingernails are clubbed. She feels for the pulse in his wrist and stares at her watch. 'About a hundred and ten beats per minute,' she says.

'The doctors told me it was two hundred last night.'

'It's still a bit quick,' she says.

I watch her go through a routine examination of his face, neck, chest and ankles, listening with her stethoscope to his lungs and heart. Steve, vast and passive as a child, lets her do everything, obedient to every request. When she finishes she thanks him and wishes him well.

'A pleasure,' he says. 'Good luck with yer studies.'

Steve looks as if he is thinking something over, making some decision, and as we turn to leave he gently reaches out a hand and touches Rebecca on the arm, his pinprick pupils are lost in eyes that bulge with emotion.

'You asked so I'll tell you,' he says in a whisper. This time he doesn't want his fellow patients to hear. 'I killed a man in Iraq and I don't even know who he was.'

Rebecca nods.

'You don't look shocked,' he says.

'I suppose I guessed that's what happens in war,' Rebecca says. She puts her hand on his arm in comfort.

I look at the monitor. Steve's heart is still cantering after his near-death experience. It will settle as the drug fades from his system. He seems a bull of a man. His body able to withstand everything he throws at it. Living to fight another day.

We thank him.

'Take care of yourself,' Rebecca says.

'Good luck with everything,' he says. 'We need good doctors.'

We turn and cross the two metres of linoleum between the beds and I approach Alastair. His heart monitor shows a textbook trace, running at textbook rate. He puts the pink newspaper down and takes off his gold specs. I ask if we can talk to and examine him.

He speaks in a soft cultured voice. 'Of course,' he says. 'Good for you.'

'What's happening in the world?' I ask, pointing at the newspaper.

'Oh, the markets are pretty chaotic,' he says. 'The Middle East as well.' He smiles. 'It's just an ordinary day.'

I ask Alastair why he's in hospital and he tells us that he began to get chest pain yesterday while he was at work.

'What were you doing?'

'Oh, umm, giving a talk to some colleagues,' he says.

'How did you feel?' I ask.

'I felt this pressure in my chest heading up into my throat, and I felt sick. Somebody said I looked pretty grey. I stopped what I was doing but the pains persisted so someone called an ambulance. But by the time I got here the pains had stopped. They did some tests and decided my coronary arteries are blocked so I should stay over and have them looked at today.'

'Was that the first time you'd felt like that?'

'Looking back I reckon for the last year I've been getting mild pains, but I just put it down to stress.'

'Where's the stress been coming from?' I ask.

He smiles. 'Oh, I have a pretty full-on job.'

I think that I recognize him from somewhere but can't quite place him.

Alastair's a non-smoker, exercises regularly, drinks alcohol in moderation and his blood pressure is OK, but there is a family history of heart disease.

'My father died of a heart attack when he was this age,' says Alastair.

'That must make this more frightening,' I say, 'but things are very different now with modern treatments.'

'Of course,' he says. 'My father smoked, and I remember him being stressed most of the time. I vowed not to be like him and –' he waves down at his lilac gown – 'here I am.'

We briefly discuss what he will undergo today. It involves passing a thin wire up from a vein in the leg, threading it up through the major blood vessels, through the chambers of the heart and then back into the arteries that clasp the heart in their grip and keep it healthy with oxygenated blood. The doctor will squirt a dye into the arteries that will highlight the areas that are narrowed by cholesterol and in those places they will slot a tiny cylinder of mesh that will expand and hold the artery open.

I ask to examine Alastair and begin the same survey of his body that Rebecca did with Steve, starting at his hands. I still have the nagging feeling that I recognize the man. I scan his white plastic hospital wristband and when I read his full name I realize I'm right. He's a senior parliamentarian who supported the 'war on terror'. The war that led to Steve killing a man.

I ask him to pull down his eyelids, open his mouth wide and stick his tongue out. I inspect and feel his hands. The backs are tanned, the palms white and soft. I check his ankles, which are slim below the muscled calves. I feel his pulse at the wrist and then in his slightly wrinkled neck, pressing gently on that intimate spot where the carotid artery pulses, his lifeblood bumping in regular heaves against my index finger. I ask him to turn to the left and watch as the blood in his largest vein flickers the skin at the base of his neck. I place my hands on his chest through the thin lilac fabric and feel the bump of the pulse in his chest. Then I listen through my stethoscope at the air sighing in and out of his lungs and then over the valves of his heart. As I'm listening I look through the window as the large river flows by with pleasure boats, barges and a police launch.

As is common for someone with furred-up coronaries the examination is entirely normal.

I thank Alastair for his time and wish him all the best. He wishes me and Rebecca luck with our studies.

We wander back over to Steve. 'Look after yourself,' I say.

'Now, Steve,' Rebecca says sternly.

'Yes,' he says.

'Are you going to take any more VanillaSky?' she asks.

'No,' Steve says.

'Really?'

'Scout's honour,' Steve growls, putting three fingers up to his temple.

'And what about other drugs?' she asks.

'No promises but I'll work on it,' Steve says. 'Just for you.'

We stand in the corner of the room to write quick notes about the cases. I think to myself it's good that those two men are getting the same care from the same doctors in the same hospital.

Behind us Steve strikes up a conversation with Alastair again. 'Would you be a fan of the Pistols then, Ally?'

Alastair puts his pink newspaper down on the blanket in front of him. 'I never really saw the point of them, to be honest.'

'Oh dear,' says Steve. 'Oh dear. A lost cause.'

The Nest

There they are. Standing in the lee of a grocery doorway, their conjoined bodies a barrier against the autumn wind as they try to light the roll-up ciggies clamped in their wrinkled mouths. She wears muted tones, a grey donkey jacket, beige khakis and desert boots. In almost comical contrast he is dressed loudly in a tweed cap, Afghan jacket, red flared trousers and golden trainers. Their clothes have the begrimed, greasy look of the committed street dweller and bulge with the many layers underneath. In a city of millions of eccentrics they don't stand out.

His arm is held firmly round the lower part of her back, like a child's round its mother's. Her arm hesitantly snakes round his back as well but higher up. He mutters sweet nothings to her as he flicks the lighter and she sucks into the low flame.

When they have successfully got the tips smouldering he turns and talks. 'We are madly in love,' Pablo says by way of introduction in a voice that seems to contain several different accents.

He speaks quietly and I can hardly hear him over the thundering traffic as we stand in the shadow of the skyscrapers, surrounded by iridescent piles of fruit from around the world: mangos, satsumas, lychees and apples. 'Aren't we, darling?'

Sonya stands a metre behind Pablo, eyes squinting up at

the ochre sky. She might be deaf for all the notice she seems to take of his words.

'We are madly in love,' he confirms. 'We were fated to be in love before we even met. The planets have decided everything for us; the planets decide everything,' he says, waving the red glowing tip of the roll-up clamped between nicotine-yellow fingers at the strange sky.

The atmosphere has an eerie yellow-orange colour and the sun shines over the vast city like a red stop light. In the canyons between the multinational corporation headquarters crowds of tourists and commuters bustle down the pavements. Red double-decker buses and black taxi cabs honk their horns in frustration at the gridlocked traffic.

'Look at the sky – this is an important day; something big will happen,' says Pablo self-importantly, and he grips Sonya's hand and looks nervous.

'The newspapers are reporting it's dust from the Sahara desert carried here on the wind,' I say.

'Do you believe everything you read?' Pablo asks.

'Not everything,' I say.

'Exactly,' he says.

Pablo is convinced that the moon is getting larger in the sky year on year and this is a sign that one day it will crash into the earth.

'Why is no one taking any notice of the moon?' he asks slyly. 'I mean, it's fairly important, right? It's going to leave a bit of a dent.' He waves his arms at the thronging street. 'All of these millions of people will have to take notice.'

'You cannot escape your fate, can you, darling?' he says to Sonya, who seems to be listening now and gives a few brittle shakes of her head. 'Take us,' he continues, 'we had no choice in the matter.'

And Pablo explains how their life together began.

They hail from a town in southern Spain from where, on a clear day, you could see across the Mediterranean to Africa. They met at school and fell in love instantly. As soon as they could, they hitch-hiked to Britain with a perfectly evolved plan for the rest of their lives: to live in a secluded cottage, grow fruit and veg in the garden, and spend the rest of their time writing and performing music. Even now they can visualize their destination.

'Small, thatched, with roses growing round the door and ivy up the walls, a vegetable patch and chickens,' says Pablo, 'but far, far away from other people.'

'We don't need them,' he continues, as we stand by the busy city thoroughfare, breathing in the diesel-laced air as an idling lorry belches out fumes. 'We never have. We are an island of two.'

The plan was born from several ingredients. In part from a desire to escape a suffocating home environment. Pablo mutters about how difficult both their families were. In part from a book one of them had read about William Wordsworth; neither could now remember which of them had read it, Pablo said. And, reading between the lines, in part from their refusal to settle to any work that was laid in front of them.

Pablo, a budding poet, would write the songs, and Sonya would sing.

'She still has a beautiful voice,' says Pablo, 'like a linnet.'

Sonya turns from where she's been rooting in a grimy

shopping trolley, returning the pouch of tobacco, and stares straight ahead of her with penetrating hazel eyes.

'Do you want to say something, Sonya?' I ask.

Pablo reaches up and puts his hand over her mouth. 'She doesn't need to,' he says.

I stare at him coldly. 'Sonya?' I say.

Pablo takes his hand down until it's hovering awkwardly in mid-air, halfway from her mouth to its natural resting position by his side. In their frozen position they look like a pair of mime artists.

'Do you want to say something, Sonya?' I repeat.

Sonya shakes her head.

We stand in silence for a while.

'My Sonya,' Pablo says, and then mutters something else that is drowned out by the squealing brakes of a bus.

They arrived at Dover with a six-string guitar, some clothes, books and a little money, then made their way further inland. Not much music had been made as far as I could tell. The guitar was sold early on. They did a few odd jobs, but could never stick at anything – or at least Pablo couldn't stick at anything and he wouldn't let Sonya try. He was a few years older than she was. It seemed he was always the dominant partner. Bar a few short interludes, they had been living rough ever since they arrived.

'And how long ago did you come to Britain?' I ask.

'Ooooh, something like forty years,' says Pablo, swivelling his creased neck to his partner, and fixing a loving pair of amber eyes on her. 'Gosh, aren't we getting old, darling?'

For the last ten years or so they have lived on the edge of an industrial estate directly under the flight path of the international airport in a sort of nest, woven from branches, leaves and plastic bags, in a thicket of trees. A scraggly blue tarpaulin knotted in the upper branches keeps off most of the rain. In the day they wander into the heart of the city.

They get their nutrition from soup kitchens and bin-diving, though they are easily intimidated from the choicest pickings by other more territorial rough sleepers. For money they sometimes get plugged into the benefits system, but more often rely on handouts on the street.

'There's more money in homelessness than busking,' observes Pablo.

They smoke like chimneys but that is their only vice. Despite the failure of their plan to bear fruit they retain a romantic view of their circumstances, or so Pablo claims.

'People think it's safer locked up indoors,' Pablo tells me. 'But it isn't. The risk of fire or violence is much greater indoors than outside. Outside you can see the danger coming from far away.'

He pats Sonya on the arm. 'She doesn't sleep much. She's a great lookout.'

I look at Sonya's beautiful wrinkled face. High cheek-bones. Greasy grey hair pulled back in a bun.

'You rely on Sonya a lot, don't you, Pablo?' I say.

'Oh yes.'

She smiles shyly.

'Do you still write poetry?' I ask him.

'I sometimes make up poems and I tell them to Sonya. I realized a long time ago she is the only audience I need.'

'Have you been together this entire time,' I ask, 'these four decades on the street?'

A dark cloud crosses Pablo's face. Sonya remains impassive.

'We had a short break a while back,' says Pablo, cast down into himself. 'I can't bear to think about it; it was hell.'

Later, at a clinic for rough sleepers, the circumstances of Pablo's and Sonya's short break from each other are explained to me. As they got older and health problems emerged, physical and mental, the couple were forced to turn up more often at the clinic to get help. While there it didn't go unnoticed by the medical staff that some of Pablo's eccentricities bordered on the delusional, including his jealousy towards Sonya. Nor was it missed that he was exceedingly domineering in their interactions. There was the talking for both of them, the raising of his hand to cover her mouth when she looked as if she might say something, and on the occasions when doctors asked him to leave so they could speak to Sonya alone he would get extremely upset – tearful and angry – such that Sonya always capitulated immediately and said she preferred to talk about things in front of him.

The doctors began to wonder how deep the coercion might run. After all there was no one else to monitor things, no one else for Sonya or Pablo to confide in, no parents or children or friends or colleagues. They really were an island of two. And what was happening on this island? Did Sonya even want to be on it? Had she ever? The horrible thought that Sonya might have spent her whole adult life friendless, family-less, jobless and on the street because of this man's psychological abuse began to worry the doctors. They arranged for a gynaecological check at the surgery and demanded that Pablo absent himself. Tearfully he acceded and removed himself to the waiting room on the other side of the five-centimetre thick door. With him banished the doctor admitted to Sonya that they just wanted to hear her side of things without Pablo in the room, just wanted to hear her speak freely.

At first she insisted that everything was fine. Pablo treated her well. She was happy with her life. They were in love.

The doctor explained their concerns. 'There are hostels,' he remembered telling her. 'You could sleep indoors, have a shower. You don't need to be on the street.'

'Would we be together there?' she asked suddenly, looking the doctor in the eyes.

'You could be,' the doctor said.

Sonya's eyes cast down.

'Or you could be apart.'

Sonya nods as she thinks this over.

'You don't have to be together if you don't want to be.'

Later, when Pablo comes back into the room, he is wild-eyed and suspicious.

'Sonya has some problems down below that we need to keep an eye on,' the doctor says.

He was not happy to hear this news at all.

It took a while for things to be arranged. Eventually it was agreed that the couple should be taken into a psychiatric hospital for assessment of their mental health. This necessarily meant they would be split up on to separate single-sex locked wards.

Pablo was furious. 'We've been together forty years. I'll kill myself.'

When she was an inpatient the psychiatrists quickly decided that Sonya was depressed and that she had been coerced over the years into a lifestyle not of her own choosing. Once she felt safe and secure away from him she expressed a desire to be apart from Pablo and they discharged her after a few days to a women's hostel. She had a room, a bed and running water for the first time in years. She started eating regular meals, washing every day, wearing clean clothes. After a while she borrowed a fellow resident's make-up, then she had her hair cut in a bob. She got a job working in a dry-cleaner's. She began to open up to people, pass the time of day, ask them about their lives. She seemed happier to the doctors, and looked like a different person, though she was always worried about how Pablo was managing without her.

Pablo was also discharged after the psychiatrists decided that he had deep-rooted personality issues relating to attachment and narcissism that would not be fixed by medication or an inpatient stay. He rejected the offer of a course of counselling to dig into these psychological problems. He was offered a room in a hostel but preferred to return to the empty nest. He spent most of his time looking for Sonya but no one would tell him where she was.

One day, after six months had elapsed, Sonya ran into Pablo in the street. That day she returned to the nest. Weeks later, when the doctors discovered what had happened, they arranged another gynaecological appointment to see her alone and find out what was going on, Pablo sitting a few metres away through five centimetres of door.

'All the time I wanted to run into him,' she said, her voice louder than they had heard it before. 'In a city this big it must have been fate. I couldn't go on without him. We were meant to be together.'

*

On the street, under the orange sky, invisible Saharan sand filling the air, still sheltering in the lee of the grocery doorway, I cannot get Pablo and Sonya apart.

So I ask Sonya directly, 'Do you have any control over your life?'

Pablo stands next to her angrily; he has taken the pouch of tobacco out of the grimy shopping trolley and starts rolling two tight cigarettes.

Sonya looks away and doesn't answer.

'You should have,' I say. 'Don't you think so, Pablo? Sonya should be able to make decisions for herself.'

Sonya doesn't speak.

'She loves me and I love her,' he says. 'It's beyond her control, beyond mine.'

I try again. 'Wouldn't you rather be off the street, Sonya, in a hostel?'

'It's safer out here,' Pablo says.

I look at Sonya, her wrinkled face still handsome, still noble. Fine lips. Sharp brown eyes set deep in the creases of the sockets.

'Why do you think Pablo loves you so much?' I ask, hoping that he will want to hear what she has to say.

Pablo goes to put his hand up towards her mouth then holds back. The city crowds stream past under the forbidding sky. The traffic in the gridlocked street honks and squeals.

'He needs me,' she says finally with a hint of an accent, that Spanish childhood still bobbing on the waves of the words.

Pablo looks satisfied, but I am unsure which question she has answered. The shopkeeper comes out and picks two of each of the fruits in the nearby boxes – two apples, two lychees, two satsumas, two mangos – places them in a paper bag and offers it to them. Pablo bows low in thanks and takes the fruit.

'Do you still sing, Sonya?' I ask.

She doesn't say anything but tears spring to her eyes.

Pablo looks on proudly. 'She has a beautiful voice,' he says.

Royal Oak

I only get a look at Dave's eyes once.

I see him every so often when I'm on call, to tinker with his drugs, to relieve his pain or to shed some of the fluid in which he is drowning, and on every occasion his eyes are closed. Whether with pain, opiates or a wish to close out the outside world, the lids are always down. At first I assume he is asleep but whenever I arrive at his bedside and dutifully report what I am about to do and seek his consent, he always answers me.

He looks like a massive pasty egg with a bushy beard, sweat-slicked hair and spectacles slipping down his shiny nose. His belly – filled with fluid, tight as a drum – protrudes through the diamond-shaped gaps in his pyjama top. He has stubby salt-and-pepper eyelashes. His eyelids twitch minutely.

He sits night and day in an armchair by his neatly made-up bed occasionally grunting, farting or shifting but otherwise immobile. Sitting out in a chair is more comfortable because if he lies down his abdomen presses painfully on his lungs and stomach and his lungs fill with fluid, making him breathless.

And the armchair seems to perfectly reflect a life hovering perpetually on the border between wake and sleep. He has no appetite for meals, doesn't want to wash or change clothes, doesn't want to listen to the radio, doesn't open his eyes long enough to register day and night. And which of us would bother with these life rituals while waiting to die?

Decades of heavy boozing have made Dave's liver inflamed and then fibrosed. Instead of a large sponge that can process toxins, fats and nutrients it is now a hardened shrivelled leathery version of itself, struggling with its most basic functions. It is failing irrevocably now and is no longer producing protein, and with less protein in the bloodstream the fluid leaks all over the place, into his flesh, into his abdomen and into his lungs.

'I was told you want more pain medication?'

'Yeahhhh,' he half growls, eyes firmly shut. 'More medication'd be good.'

'OK,' I say. 'Let's increase the morphine then.' I scribble on the chart.

'I'd murder a pint,' Dave says, eyes still closed.

With the lack of facial movement I can't work out if he's joking. He seems more just to be expressing the natural thought.

'Not available, Dave,' I say.

'Yeahhh,' he growls acceptingly. 'Whisky then?'

'None of that either.'

'Bacardi?'

And so it goes on. All the time Dave's eyes stay shut.

A few weeks later I'm a little surprised to see him still on the duty list. I thought he would be dead by now. He needs a replacement tube stuck into his vein to administer the meds to help shed the fluid and no one has been able to do it. Without the medication his lungs will fill up with fluid more quickly.

He's still in the same chair, eyes still firmly shut, looking even more ghastly. Now the fluid seems to be oozing from his skin, slicking his hair, face and body with an oily sheen, marinading him. I warn him about what I'm going to do, unsure if he is awake.

As usual he replies. 'You carry on,' he growls, eyes closed.

I poke the needle and find a vein. His face doesn't even exhibit a twitch.

'Success,' I say as strange thin yellowy-purple blood climbs the needle.

Dave mutters something incoherent.

Why should he care if this works or not? I tape the cannula down to his arm, but the adhesive won't stick to the slick of fluid coating his skin. I watch as the pink cannula begins to float out of his vein, carried on the tide of the fluid leaving his body. I use my finger to hold it in place and fashion a harness from the tape and tie it round and round his arm as a kind of mooring to hold the tiny plastic vessel in place. It works just long enough for me to start tidying everything away, but then the tape slithers off his arm.

After several similar efforts I say, 'I'm sorry, Dave. I don't think this is going to work.'

'Don't worry,' he grunts.

I let the cannula leap out of his body and tidy things up. There's little else to do. There's no way we're going to get any of these simple bedside lines to stay in his body, and it's already been decided we're not going to try the more complex lines. Dave is for ward care only. Without the medication he is just likely to die a bit quicker, that's all.

'Is there someone I can get you, Dave, family, a friend, a priest?'

'I'd like to get out of here to get a drink,' he grunts, eyes still closed.

I sit on the side of his unused bed and stare out of the window pondering his complete infatuation with booze. Jesus, you can actually see the Royal Oak from this vantage point. It's the pub where the doctors go after work to settle their nerves and exchange war stories. What was that old definition of an alcoholic, someone who drinks more than their doctor? Is this why Dave's eyes are closed? The pub is an unbearable sight – a far-off, unreachable oasis spotted by a man in the desert dying of thirst.

For a lunatic second I entertain the prospect of springing Dave for a drink. He's dying anyway. It's a free world. People on death row get a last meal, why not a last drink for Dave? Then the technical and ethical difficulties flood in. First do no harm. Getting his massive frame from chair to wheelchair. What if he dies in the pub?

'You like alcohol?' I say, deciding not to mention my idea.

'Love it,' he growls with passion. 'Always have, ever since my first drop. I love it,' he repeats, eyes still closed, seemingly off in some booze-soaked memory. With me but also not with me.

What will probably kill Dave are the levels of urea in his blood. These will climb and climb until they make his brain swell and the bits of his brain that make him breathe stop functioning. Either that or an infection will sweep through his body with its ruined immune system. Or the fluid will drown him or put too much pressure on his heart so he has a heart attack. Or his kidneys will stop functioning and the levels of salinity in his blood will dive and so on and so forth.

But what use is this knowledge set against the man's drive to drink?

'What work did you do?' I ask.

'Joiner,' he answers immediately. He's here all right. Just has his eyes closed. 'Long time ago,' he adds.

'What kind of things did you make?'

'Doors, tables, cupboards, you know.' He sounds irritated at the question.

'Did you like it?'

'Was a job,' he says.

'Have you got any family?'

'Naaah.'

'Ever married?'

'Yeahhh.' He lets out a deep sigh, and for a moment I think it's the emotion of what we are talking about, though he also seems to be in some physical pain, and shifting a little in his chair seems to fix the problem.

'Bitch left me,' he grunts. 'Couldn't take the drinking.'

'Did your parents drink?'

'Yeah,' he says. 'Plenty.'

I look at his drawn sweat-smeared face, the eyes closed.

I think of the meetings I've sat in where they discuss who gets the liver transplants; it's all done on a case by case, liver by liver basis. A task of Solomon-like wisdom. Factors include the reasons why the liver has been ruined, the age and general health of the patient, their mental state. Low on the list of priorities are the chronic alcoholics. If there are livers to spare for them, they have to show their commitment to this precious new organ, this complex surgery, a lifetime of medical care by undergoing psychological treatment and quitting booze for some specific length of time without relapse.

'Did you ever try to stop?' I ask. 'I know it's difficult to stop.'

'Once,' Dave says, 'A mistake. And I realized it was the only thing I truly love.'

His eyelids roll up to reveal eyes as yellow as egg yolks. He looks at me, and the look on his sodden face spells triumph.

Walking

Mrs Musa is detained for walking through a large park. Not unusual in itself. There are hundreds of city dwellers marching past the boating lake on their way to work or to shop, parents pushing babies in buggies, tourists ambling, people talking on phones, listening to music, clutching coffee. But something about the way Mrs Musa does it, the hunted look on her face, her dishevelled appearance, her bare feet on frosty ground in the dead of winter, something makes the police car winding slowly through the park stop and two officers get out to talk to her.

At this approach Mrs Musa makes a dash for it, fear in her eyes. She's out of shape, and older, and it doesn't take the police long to catch up. When they do Mrs Musa goes very quiet and still like a rabbit caught in headlights. They escort her back to the car. She doesn't tell them her name and they cannot find any ID on her. Eventually back at the station someone makes a connection with a call logged from her family that morning to say their mother, a Nigerian woman fitting Mrs Musa's description, had gone missing.

When the police say they will take her back home Mrs Musa gets agitated and starts screaming. So they take her to a 136 Suite in the local A & E department for assessment. Mrs Musa is incoherent and distraught, and the duty psychiatrist prescribes her a regular sedative and tables her for an inpatient psychiatric bed for assessment.

*

By the time I meet Mrs Musa on Larch Ward in the psychiatric hospital she has spent two days in the general hospital waiting for a bed to become available. In that time she made several attempts to walk off the ward.

The paperwork I read in the small doctor's office tells the story of the day she went missing. Her daughter had returned from the shops to find their suburban house empty. She rang her brother who drove around the local area trying to locate her, but when that failed they called the police. I can see that Mrs Musa's record shows no medical problems to speak of until a year previously when she had attended her GP. They had diagnosed low mood, prescribed an antidepressant and asked her to return for a follow-up appointment, which she did not do.

I assess Mrs Musa, with her two adult children, in a quiet glass-walled room giving out on to a frosty garden. Although it's only four in the afternoon, dusk is falling. A lone robin hops up and down in the blue light. Its yammering beak silently cheeps a territorial song through the thick glass walls. Through a glass door we can see into an anteroom where Mrs Musa's much younger son, Osinachi, is patiently sitting and reading a book with a nurse.

The patient sits an arm's length away round the oval oak table from me. She is dressed in baggy tracksuit trousers and an untucked pink shirt with a navy woollen jumper. Her posture is unnaturally still. She is drawn in on herself with arms crossed and eyes cast down. There are patches of grey in her dishevelled black tight curled hair. Her black skin has a sheen of sweat. Flecks of spittle dance at the corner of her mouth. Her brown eyes are bloodshot. She looks a decade older than her fifty-eight years.

Mrs Musa's adult daughter and son are smartly dressed and groomed in stark contrast to their odoriferous mother.

The daughter, Zainab, sits just behind her mother. She has a delicate bone structure and piercing light brown eyes. She is quiet and watchful. Her younger brother, Adam, sits on the other side of the table – tall, thin, trim beard, brown eyes, a small crystal crescent adorning one ear. He seems hostile.

'No one at the hospital was able to tell us what was going on. No one is helping us. No one is helping our mother. We're here to make sure she's looked after properly.' He looks angry and afraid. 'This is not who she is. She's a great mother. She always worked hard for us. It's horrible seeing her like this.'

'I don't think they knew what was going on at the hospital,' I say, 'and she's lucky to have your support. We'll get to the bottom of things here.'

But after a while I'm beginning to doubt my own words. Mrs Musa just will not or cannot answer any of my questions. How she is feeling, how she is sleeping, how does she find the food, does she know where she is?

After each question we sit in complete silence. Mrs Musa is trembling, wrapped tightly in her own arms. It's not even clear that she is hearing what I am saying.

Adam impatiently fiddles with his earring. Zainab is still. The robin silently hops and chirps outside.

'Mrs Musa, do you understand me?'

'Mrs Musa, do you feel safe here?'

'Do you mind if I ask your children some questions?'

She still says nothing so I turn to them. 'How long has your mother been like this?'

I'm not sure if I imagine it but both of them suddenly look fearful. I let the question hang there but they don't answer.

'What was she like . . . before?' I say.

'Very different,' Adam says finally.

'Please tell me.'

'She was full of energy,' Adam says eventually. 'Our dad died when we were young and she had to get work. She did different jobs, cook, cleaner, bus driver, often two at the same time. She didn't want us to miss out because of Dad, so she even taught us how to play football. She pushed us to be good at everything. She was the boss. She loved cooking, singing Nigerian music. She was happy.'

I look at Mrs Musa as this is said about her. She seems to shudder but her brown eyes don't even blink. I try to see the person Adam is describing. To mentally clean her up, dress her smartly, relax her, animate her, give her confidence, a voice.

Darkness is falling and the glass walls are becoming mirrors, mixing dark shadows from outside with our reflections.

'I like music too, Mrs Musa,' I say. 'Who do you like to listen to?'

But she doesn't appear to hear me.

'Do you like Fela Kuti?' I ask, referencing the only Nigerian singer I know. But Mrs Musa seems just as far away.

'What does she do now?' I ask her children.

'She just sits in her chair all day and all night,' says Adam.

'Just sits,' I repeat.

'Doesn't go to bed. Hardly eats anything. Hardly speaks,' he continues.

Zainab wipes a tear from her eye.

'It's been going on too long . . .' Adam says angrily.

'How long?' I ask.

There's a long pause and then, very reluctantly, Adam replies. 'About four years.'

We sit in silence. I try not to show my surprise. Zainab looks shocked by the revelation coming out. *Four years*, I think. *Four years. Poor woman.*

Mrs Musa trembles. A bubble of spit develops at the corner of her mouth then pops.

'Four years?' I say. 'Mrs Musa, that sounds very difficult.'

Her disrepair seems deeper now I know how long it's been going on. Her distance makes more sense. She sits there, eyes bulging, no acknowledgement of what we're talking about.

'We tried to look after her ourselves,' Adam says. 'Zainab did everything for her, cooking, washing. I got a better-paying job to cover her income. We both looked after Osi.' He points through the glass door at the child sitting with the nurse. 'But she just got more and more withdrawn. Eventually she moved out of her bedroom and just sat downstairs all day and all night.'

Adam sounds defensive. But it seems entirely natural. They are a private, close-knit family. 'We thought that was best for her, to be looked after by her family. That's how we do it in our culture.'

Through the glass door their young half-brother Osinachi is pointing at a picture in the book and smiling at the nurse.

'Did anything happen four years ago?' I ask.

Zainab seems to freeze but Adam answers. 'She stopped working. She stopped seeing her friends. Wouldn't go out.'

'I mean, did anything happen to her that could explain her change in behaviour?'

But Adam seems not to hear the question. 'She was just different.'

There's something they're not telling me, I feel. But I decide to come back to it later.

'Why did you end up taking her to the GP?'

'She began walking,' says Adam.

'Walking?'

'Yes, a few months back she left the house and didn't come back. She'd walked off ten miles. I had to track her down and pick her up in the car. After that she began to go off walking most days.'

'Was she going somewhere?' I ask.

'No,' Adam looks at me bewildered, 'just seemed to be walking in random directions. Every time I'd have to drive out and find her and pick her up. She was reluctant to get into the car, but eventually I could persuade her.'

Adam rubs his carefully trimmed stubble with a forefinger and looks saddened by the memory. 'We took her to the GP but they didn't seem to know what to do, just stuck her on antidepressants.'

'Did the medication help?'

'Not really,' he says. 'So instead we began locking the door.'

In the anteroom Osinachi and the nurse are patiently building a neat tower of finger-length wooden blocks. It's fully dark outside now. The garden and the robin have disappeared. We are now sitting in a reflective box. The strip lights are golden bars bouncing back off the glass walls. The walls depict several Adams, several Zainabs, several Mrs Musas. I watch our reflections in their gilded cage, the clock ticking down the seconds until the rest of us leave and Mrs Musa remains.

I think of her locked in her own home, a prisoner for her own protection. Is this why Zainab looks so guilty? Will we do the same to her here? Imprison her because walking in a park in bare feet looks odd? I need to get inside her somehow, get her to trust us, to open up.

I turn back to Mrs Musa. 'How are you feeling?'

No answer. She remains wrapped and cocooned in herself.

'Do you feel safe?' I ask again. No words, but there's a flicker of her bloodshot eyes, a look from the befuddlement of her sedated mind that says no.

And then Zainab leans in from behind her and puts her hand softly on her shoulder. 'Mum, you're safe here. You can talk,' she says, and leaves her hand there.

Tears well in Mrs Musa's eyes and dribble down her cheeks and lips and into her mouth. We sit in silence and watch her emotion leak out.

'What is frightening you?' I ask finally.

Slowly, for the first time, she unlocks her arms from their tight self-embrace and extends them forward, hands trembling, and turns her palms to face the ceiling.

'What is it?' I ask.

The mumbled words are barely audible. 'I'm not safe.'

'What is the threat?' I say, reaching out a hand to her.

She lets me take her hand in mine. It's moist with sweat. I try a new gambit.

'Sometimes when people are feeling distressed they hear things or see things that other people can't. Have you ever had any experiences like that?'

She flinches but doesn't withdraw her hand. She looks directly at me for the first time, eyes bulging, her fear welling out from behind the veil of sedation. There's a look of hope on her face, as if perhaps I might just understand her. I hold her sweating palm in my grip.

'The bird,' she says.

'Tell me . . .'

'I saw it today.'

'Where?'

'At home. It's at home.'

'Is there a bird at home?' I ask her children.

They look confused and shake their heads.

'No,' says Zainab.

'How long has this bird been in your house?' I ask Mrs Musa.

She looks at me with her bloodshot eyes. 'A long time.'

'It's real, is it?'

Mrs Musa nods.

'What kind of bird is it?' I ask.

Mrs Musa flinches. 'A vulture.'

'You never mentioned that, Mum,' Adam says.

'What does it do?'

'It waits.' Mrs Musa waves her free hand across her own head, the other still gripping mine. Quietly but firmly she makes the syllables distinct. 'It's waiting.'

'For what?'

'For me to die.'

'Why?'

She shakes her head, lips tightly pressed shut, then she pulls her hand away from mine and uses it to wrap herself up in her arms again.

'Is that why you tried to leave home?' I ask.

Mrs Musa doesn't speak. We sit in silence for a minute.

'Is the vulture here now?' I ask.

'No,' Mrs Musa says.

'You're safe here,' I say. 'It can't hurt you.'

She nods as if to herself.

'Mrs Musa, did anything happen four years ago?' I ask.

Adam tenses, as if worried about what his mother might say.

'It's OK,' Zainab says, putting her other hand on her mother's arm and rubbing it.

'Zay,' her brother Adam says, a warning tone in his voice.

'Mum needs our help,' Zainab says. 'They need to know.'

She has a strong gentle voice. She turns a fierce gaze on me. Her brown eyes flash. 'Ten years ago Mum remarried and had Osi –' she points through the glass door at the boy who is carefully removing one wooden block from the lower reaches of the tower, making sure it doesn't tumble down. 'Mum was pretty old to have a baby and things got bad with my stepfather almost straight away and he left and went home to Nigeria. Four years ago he came over to visit Osi and took him back to Nigeria with him.'

'He kidnapped him,' Adam cuts in dully.

'Mum went out to try to get him back,' Zainab continues.

She puts an arm round her shoulders. 'But the family kidnapped her too. They hurt her. They treated her very badly.'

Mrs Musa looks frozen to the spot.

'It's different out there. The rules are different,' Zainab continues.

I look at Adam. His face has gone pale and tears tumble silently down his face.

We sit surrounded by the multiple glassy reflections of ourselves. In the anteroom Osi and the nurse have pulled out several wooden blocks and the tower is beginning to look precarious.

I think about the bird that Mrs Musa has been living with, sitting and waiting. Zainab must be following the same train of thought. She puts her hand on her mother's shoulder again. 'Mum told me that one day, after weeks of being imprisoned, she escaped to try to get help. She walked and walked and walked along the highway. She said there were vultures circling in the sky and she thought she would collapse and they would eat her. Eventually she got tired and the kidnappers caught up with her . . .' Her story tails off.

'How did she escape?' I ask.

Adam dries his tears with his sleeve. His face is pinched and he speaks in a low tight voice. 'We got in contact with a businessman out in that province and paid money, a lot of money. He negotiated a ransom to get Mum and Osi back and we paid it.

'When they got back Mum was very upset, very angry with herself. At first she refused to tell us what had happened but eventually she did. We looked after her but she couldn't go back to work, couldn't bear to see anyone apart from us in the home, and gradually she just got worse and worse.'

'She'd always prided herself on keeping us safe,' Zainab says softly. 'The world she'd tried to build was broken.'

Mrs Musa sits wrapped up in her own arms. She makes no sign that she has heard what we have been saying. The flecks of spit dance on the fringes of her cheeks. She has spent four years buried deep beneath humiliation and fear – unable to protect her son, unable to be a mother. How long ago had the hallucinations started?

'You did your best,' Zainab says softly to her mother. 'You are so brave.'

'Mum,' Adam says, 'were you walking to get away from this, this vulture?'

Mrs Musa's whole body shudders.

Adam closes his eyes and shakes his head. 'Part of me always felt like I was doing the wrong thing when I brought her back home.' He stands up and walks behind his mother and puts his arms round her neck and kisses her on her head. 'I'm sorry, Mum.'

Through the glass door in the anteroom Osi cautiously pulls out another wooden block. Somehow the tower remains upright.

In my mind's eye I see vast green mountains. Vultures wheeling in the thermals. A long empty highway. Freedom.

I think of Mrs Musa walking along the highway in Nigeria, walking down the suburban streets, walking by the boating lake a few days ago, trying to escape. She's been locked up once in Nigeria, then by her family, and now by us. How will we set her free?

The End

On a Monday evening in the run-up to Christmas a woman in her late fifties with a shock of grey hair is brought to the hospital feverish and gasping for breath. After giving her high-flow oxygen through a mask we get an X-ray done, which shows one lung is half filled with fluid, so we cut a hole between her ribs and insert a tube as thick as a thumb to drain the fluid off. We drip high doses of antibiotics straight into her veins and ask the night team to keep an eye on her before heading home.

On Tuesday morning I find Diana in a side room in a far-flung reach of the hospital. Through the window the pale wintry light paints the city a deep grey. A large brown river cuts through the middle, flowing silently past.

Her breathing is calmer now and she only requires a trickle of oxygen delivered by small rubber prongs that sit snugly in her nostrils. Her face is gaunt, and hanging from a string round her neck is a beautiful depiction of a small silver moon complete with seas and craters. The tube emerging from her chest curls elegantly into a tank of pink water next to her bed, which bubbles with her every breath.

'How much have you removed from the lung?' Diana asks in a low, exhausted voice.

I look at the blood-stained fluid at the bottom of the tank. 'About a litre and a half,' I say.

'I'm so grateful to be able to breathe,' she says. 'Yesterday it felt as if I was drowning.'

'I'm glad you're feeling better,' I say.

'It sounds as if I have an infection,' she adds.

'It seems like it,' I say, 'but if you've got the energy it'd be useful to hear what's been going on so we can work that out. Do you feel strong enough to talk?'

'Of course,' she says, and with some physical effort she tells me her story. That she'd been feeling tired for a few months and losing weight. She went to her GP a month back who ran blood tests that came back normal. The symptoms were put down to stress because there's a lot of that in her job in the university department. Then she went on a field trip overseas to help with the construction of a new telescope. She began to feel short of breath out there and put this down to the altitude. But on her return just a few days ago she began coughing up green phlegm and the breathlessness got worse.

'I felt as if I was running to catch a train even when I was sitting down. Thankfully you intervened, and today I feel as if I've caught the train and been sitting down for a few minutes to recover my breath as it pulls out of the station.'

As I tie a rubber tourniquet round Diana's arm and wipe the bulging vein with alcohol she describes the telescope she is working on. It will be able to see far into the universe and far back almost to the beginnings of time.

'If we can see back to the beginning,' she says, 'it may help us understand where it will end.'

'Seriously?' I say. 'I had no idea we could do that.'

She laughs and then starts coughing and choking and has to recover herself. 'I suppose you doctors spend all your time looking inwards. And maybe I've spent too long looking far outwards.'

I stick a needle in her veins and her ruby-coloured blood is sucked into the vacuum tubes.

'Will that tell us if I'm getting better?' she asks.

'It'll help,' I say, 'though how you're feeling is a more useful guide.'

'Honestly? I feel a million times better,' she says. 'I'm on the mend.'

The acrid water tank bubbles away at her side.

'Good,' I say.

'I've got so much work to do,' she says, her mind returning to the telescope. 'I must speak to the department about managing the work while I'm in here.'

On Wednesday morning I find Diana deep in conversation with a gentle-looking man. They are talking about a dog. He introduces himself as Jonathan, her husband.

He has brought a bright sprig of flowering cherry from their garden, which sits in a plastic water jug next to her bed.

I perch on the side of Diana's bed and break the news that we've looked at the lung fluid under a microscope and it has shown cancerous cells.

Diana's head slumps a little on hearing the news. Jonathan grips her hand tightly and mutters something in her ear.

'I half expected it,' she says eventually. 'I guess I need to let the department know; they'll probably have to postpone my next trip.'

I explain that Diana will need a CT scan this afternoon and a blood transfusion in the meantime as her red cell count shows she is anaemic.

The water tank at her side bubbles away with each breath. I can see that another half-litre of claggy blood-stained fluid has been pushed out of her chest overnight.

'Why has the red cell count dropped?' Jonathan asks.

'It's probably a combination of things,' I say. 'The infected lung will have become raw so blood vessels will have bled into it, and –' I stop and look at them frankly – 'and the cancer can affect the ability of the bone marrow to create new red blood cells, and it can damage the existing ones too.'

'What kind of cancer is it going to be?' asks Diana. 'I smoked a bit of pot when I was younger. Do you remember?' she asks Jonathan.

He smiles. 'I don't think Doctor T wants to hear about our misspent youth.'

'At some point I'd love to hear about your misspent youth,' I say, 'but I doubt the pot has anything to do with it, and we do really need the CT scan and maybe a biopsy before we can tell you what type of cancer it is.'

While I hang up the bag of blood and connect it to Diana, Jonathan tells her that the previous evening the family golden retriever jumped into the stream that snakes through their back garden and got stuck.

'I actually fell in while I was getting him out,' he says. 'It was freezing.'

'I'm glad you did that,' Diana says, a smile lighting up her angular face. 'It's good to know you love him enough to fall in.'

'I didn't do it on purpose,' Jonathan says. 'Next time I'll call the fire brigade.'

That afternoon Diana has a whole-body CT scan. Later, on a portable computer, I scroll through the images that show little spiky clumps of abnormal tissue lighting up like stars within the black space of the lung.

Looking at Diana lying in bed she seems to be breathing a bit more shallowly and I can see that the oxygen level delivered through the nasal prongs has been increased. I explain that a sample of the abnormal tissue has been taken to the lab and will be cut, stained and placed between glass slides and looked at under a microscope. Only then will we know what exactly is going on and what treatment might be available.

'And when will that be?' Jonathan asks. There's an edge in his calm voice.

'One or two days,' I say.

'OK,' Jonathan says, trying to hide his fears.

Diana is keen to tell me about a museum she went to on her recent field trip, high up in the mountains, which was full of ancient artefacts left by the native people.

'It almost never rains up there so the things are beautifully preserved. Their pots, their clothes, their mummified ancestors. They had temples in the mountains where they worshipped the sun. They would smoke herbs that made them hallucinate before going to the temples to get closer to their gods. A bit like what we're doing with our telescope.'

'Without the drugs presumably,' Jonathan adds, 'otherwise I'd have to report you to the university authorities.'

Diana starts laughing, then coughing and puts some tissue to her mouth. When she pulls it away we can see the phlegm is jade-coloured with streaks of fresh ruby blood.

'Damn this chest,' she says, unable to suppress her emotions.

*

On Thursday morning I arrive early to do another blood test. Through the window the tidal river is flowing against gravity, up and away from the sea. The water tank by the bed bubbles away with each breath. Diana looks exhausted and pale, her eyes sunken. She is wincing with pain from the chest drain.

'Have you had a difficult night?' I ask.

'To be honest I feel dreadful,' Diana says. 'Everything hurts. Speaking, breathing, eating, going to the loo. The tube site is a bit sore,' she says in a quiet voice, pointing to her side, 'but they gave me some of that morphine you prescribed.'

'Oh good,' I say.

'It dealt with the pain but it gave me funny dreams. I thought I was in the garden back at home and I'd been stung by a bee, and then the sting became a hole and then the bee got inside me.'

'That's no good,' I say.

'It was actually quite a relief to wake up,' she says, 'for a moment at least.'

We leave that thought hanging.

'Have you been home since we last saw you, Doctor Templeton?' Jonathan asks me, changing the subject.

'I slept in the mess,' I say, smoothing my shirt in a vain attempt to get rid of the wrinkles. 'Our firm is on-call this week, so we'll be around a lot.'

'So we're your family for the week,' he says with a twinkle. 'Can I get you a cup of coffee?'

'Thank you, but I'm fine,' I say. 'How's the breathing today, Diana?'

'Better,' she says bravely, 'I suppose that's the transfusion.'

I bleed her again and we chat about their three grown-up children and the grandchildren, and how proud she is of all of them. How the kids have all turned out differently to how she expected, how they're on loan to you, not owned. How they've all gone into fields completely removed from her own.

'But Lucy's a teacher,' says Jonathan, 'just like you.'

'She teaches English lit,' says Diana. 'She's interested in people and all that messy stuff, I'm interested in physics and chemistry, the hard rules of life and the universe.'

'It's still teaching,' says Jonathan. 'Neither of you can stop yourselves. I should know; I've had to live with it. Doctor T, over the years I've had almost everything in life explained to me, often many times, from Darwinism to Dadaism,' he says, laughing, 'and what good has it done me?'

'And what do you do?' I ask.

'I'm an accountant,' he says. 'I like the security of numbers.'

'I need your help, Doctor T,' says Diana. 'Jonathan is refusing to get me a mirror so I can look at myself. Do you think that's fair given that I can't get out of bed to fetch one myself?'

Jonathan chuckles. 'I'm not refusing. I just forgot to bring it. I never was any good at packing.'

I look at Diana. Her skin, tight on her face, has a faint yellow tinge. I make a mental note to add liver-function tests to the blood panel.

'I'll ask the nurses to find one for you,' I say.

When I come back a few hours later Diana waves a small circular mirror with a pink plastic frame triumphantly.

'I can see why Jonathan didn't want me to have this. I look shrivelled up, just like those mummies I saw in the mountains.'

'You just need a good night of beauty sleep,' Jonathan says. 'Like Doctor T here.'

This elicits a throaty laugh from Diana.

'We can try a sleeping pill tonight,' I say.

'Me or you?' Diana asks and laughs again, but it hurts her chest and she has to stop. 'This is how we see into the universe,' she says, pointing at the mirror in her hand and speaking haltingly. 'Giant saucer-shaped versions of this that collect and focus the light from the stars.'

Jonathan chuckles. 'Did I mention that Diana is a teacher?'

I have more bad news to deliver. I explain that her red cell count has improved but the levels of potassium in her blood are dangerously high. We need to repeat the test, do a heart tracing, and give her some medication to reduce the potassium.

'If it's not one thing it's another,' says Jonathan, showing his frustration.

'Do what you have to do,' Diana says.

I look at Diana's raw-boned face, her slender arms; she does look like a mummy. I can see why Jonathan is concerned.

'Tell me, Doctor T, where does the potassium come from?' Diana asks.

'It's stored in each of your cells and unfortunately, as cells are getting damaged, it's raising the amount in the bloodstream.'

A beautiful smile spreads across Diana's withered face. Her teeth are large, white and regular. 'It was a rhetorical question . . .' She winces with pain at the syllabic effort then continues. 'The potassium in my body and yours comes from . . . nuclear reactions when stars explode. Just one of the complex coincidences that came together to allow . . . biological life on Earth.'

Jonathan smiles but wanly this time. 'Did we mention Diana is a teacher?' he says again.

When I come back that afternoon two of Diana's children are in the room. A pleasant pair, plucked from their busy lives, jobs, spouses, own kids, into the no-man's land, the alternate universe, of hospital.

Diana looks very pale and washed out. She is playing Scrabble with her grown-up son. Her hands shake and she fumbles the tiles. 'I can't do it,' she says, frustrated.

'Don't worry, Mum,' her son says. 'Why don't we carry on later?' He starts packing up the board.

Jonathan tells me the oncologist has been and told them she has lung cancer.

'He said it could be curable,' Jonathan says.

'He wasn't exactly clear –' Diana says, pausing halfway through the sentence to catch her breath – 'about treatment.'

I listen to her chest. The lower sections of both lungs are now quiet, without the sound of air coming in or out that you'd expect. Her oxygen levels have fallen again. I get her to sit up in bed, increase the flow of oxygen through the nasal prongs and order a portable chest X-ray to her bedside. Then I repeat the blood test to check we've successfully reduced the potassium.

Diana's daughter is explaining how a month previously her five-year-old daughter climbed to the top of an apple tree and refused to come down for dinner, preferring instead to dine on the apples.

'She seems to like high places, like her grandmother,' Jonathan says.

'That's a . . . well-brought-up . . . girl,' Diana says haltingly.

'You'll be pleased to know we got her a telescope for Christmas,' Jonathan says.

Their daughter smiles. 'I'm amazed it's taken you both this long.'

An hour later I stand in front of a computer monitor looking at the most recent X-ray with my boss, Dr Chen.

In the X-ray we can see the faint outline of Diana's gown, her body and her breasts. Grey-white in the centre of the image is Diana's spinal column and the ribcage hanging off it to either side; the silver moon pendant is transformed into a bright white circle hanging just off centre.

I pull up the X-ray from when she arrived at hospital on Monday so the two images sit side by side and we focus on the contents of the ribcage. Monday, before we started treating her, and today Thursday. In both images her heart is half submerged under fluid in the left lung, which means all the fluid that we pulled off with the chest drain has been replaced. And now in the right lung, which was pretty much clear on Monday, there is a new collection of fluid. The surface of the fluid in both lungs is concave, like the mirrors that collect the light in Diana's telescopes.

There are too many backward steps here: the infection, the anaemia, the potassium, the fluid. 'She's not going to get well enough to have the chemo, is she?' I say, frustration welling up inside me.

Dr Chen's usually cherubic face is grave.

'Someone should tell her,' I say.

'I think you're right,' he says, tapping his fingers from the right lung that was previously clear to the right lung that is now partially obscured. 'I think you're right.'

Jonathan is sitting in a chair next to the head of the bed reading to Diana from a book.

> That strain again, it had a dying fall.
> O, it came o'er my ear like the sweet sound
> That breathes upon a bank of violets.

He looks up and looks me straight in the eye. 'We were going to get Diana's father to come and visit tomorrow morning. Do you think that would be a good idea?'

'I think that would be an excellent idea,' I say, trying to sound neutral.

Diana looks at me quizzically, then relaxes her face and smiles.

We start a medication to help remove fluid via the kidneys. We open the chest drain up again and it starts draining more fluid into the bubbling water tank by the bed. We hang up another bag of blood to transfuse into her veins.

Diana asks for some water. As I'm pouring it Dr Chen walks in.

'Hi,' he says, walking up to the foot of her bed. 'Diana, how are you getting on?'

Diana perks up a bit at his presence and rotates her hand back and forth in equivocation.

'I spoke to Doctor Venables, the oncologist, about the diagnosis,' Dr Chen says. 'How are you feeling about it?'

Diana rotates her hand again and speaks slowly and so quietly it's hard to hear. 'I'm frightened . . . and . . . I feel . . . like a . . . wimp.'

'You're no wimp,' Dr Chen says. He stands there at the foot of the bed looking at Diana with his pale blue eyes.

'You're no wimp,' he repeats after what seems an eternity, looking her straight in the eyes.

'Doctor . . . Vena . . . bles . . . tells me . . . the cancer . . . is treatable,' says Diana.

'In theory,' Dr Chen says slowly. 'In theory. But, Diana, the infection and the anaemia have taken a lot out of you. An awful lot out of you.'

There is a very long pause while Dr Chen stares at her to confirm that he is telling her that this is it. This is the end.

Diana understands. Her face contorts momentarily and she closes her eyes, then she opens them again and her face relaxes. Jonathan leans in to her, tears in his eyes and takes her hands. He whispers something in her ear and they kiss.

'Are there things you need to do?' Dr Chen asks.

She thinks about this for a long time before answering. 'No . . .' she says, smiling faintly at Jonathan, 'nothing.'

Dr Chen stands at the foot of the bed. 'We will keep you comfortable,' he says.

'Thank you . . .' she says, 'for . . . being straight . . . with me.'

The next morning is Friday. It's crisp and cold outside. A tiny green plastic Christmas tree has appeared in the doctors' mess with three golden baubles hanging off at different altitudes. In the side room an orange light filters in the window. Diana seems to be rambling a bit. She starts telling me something which is either about the mummies up in the mountains again or perhaps about mothers in general. It's hard to tell.

She also seems to be in a lot of pain. I prescribe her some medications to help with distress and with pain.

'Let the nurses know if these don't work,' I tell Jonathan. 'They can always give her more.'

Later that afternoon I come to check on her and find Diana lying in bed, seemingly asleep, a pair of headphones on her head. Her father – old but sprightly-looking – is sitting with Jonathan and his three children. He has a clump of white hair above each ear, tortoiseshell glasses and a shy smile. They are conversing quietly.

'I just wanted to check Diana is comfortable,' I say to the family.

'She's been much better,' says Jonathan. 'The pain seems to be controlled.'

'She's always been brave,' Diana's father says. 'She fell off a high swing when she was a girl; she was pale as a ghost but she refused to cry. Her arm was broken in two places.'

'Stubborn's another word for it,' Diana's son says.

'I call it brave,' the elderly man says quietly. I can see the tears hovering behind the thick spectacles.

'You're right, Grandpa,' he says. 'I don't disagree.'

I check the water tank next to Diana's bed. With each shallow breath she takes bubbles rise rapidly through the water and vanish after breaking the surface. There's a new-found peace to her face, still skeletal but less strained.

Someone has brought her an old-fashioned Walkman and a cassette tape is slowly unspooling within. I see the case on the bedside table, with a picture of a snowy landscape and the legend SCHUBERT: WINTER JOURNEY. It sits next to the cards exhorting Diana to get well, the photos of her smiling grandchildren and a golden retriever, and the sprig of cherry blossom in the plastic jug of water.

The next day we aren't called to see Diana and I presume everything is fine. In the evening before I leave for home I make my way to the side-room door. I look in through the rectangle of glass. It's dark apart from a bedside lamp. Diana is sitting up in bed holding Jonathan's hand, eyes closed. He is reading to her from a book.

On Sunday morning I knock on the door and enter the room. Diana lies in bed, peacefully, the moon pendant round her neck with its seas and craters. The water tank has been detached and is now sitting silent and still in a corner of the room. Through the window a barge is silently travelling upriver, against the flow. Jonathan sits in silence with the children. Their eyes are red raw.

I tell them how sorry I am and sorry that it all happened so quickly.

Jonathan stands and gives me a hug. I feel his body warm through our clothes.

'It was a privilege to have met her,' I say. 'She was amazing.'

'She was,' Jonathan says.

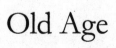

Old Age

Air Crash

'You may know a lot about bones, Mr Maloney, but you are not my mother!'

The voice emanating from the blue curtain is strong, low, clipped and confident. I slip in round the side to rejoin the afternoon orthopaedic ward round in the A & E cubicle. I can see Mr Maloney, the consultant surgeon, a former rugby prop, towering over a thick-set lady with curly hair and spectacles, lying in the bed, the covers pulled aside to reveal her right leg, which is not moving much. She adjusts her position in the bed, wincing as she does so, and looks up sternly at Mr Maloney.

'My mother was always telling me what to do, and most of the time she was wrong,' she says.

'Mrs Stone,' says Mr Maloney in his Galway brogue with a grin, 'I am just explaining that in my opinion a conservative approach is best.'

'Best for whom, Mr Maloney? Best for whom? You have already told me that without the operation I may not get the proper function at the hip. That means I will not be able to fly again . . .'

'You will be able to fly,' Mr Maloney says, 'but perhaps not as the pilot.'

She tilts her head back and glares at him through the correct portion of her thick-rimmed multifocal spectacles. 'As my father would have said, "That, young man, is not flying."'

Mr Maloney nods thoughtfully as if to acknowledge her point, then speaks slowly and clearly. 'Mrs Stone, this is a complex fracture in a site where you've already had a prosthesis and operations are not risk free. If we operate, there's a risk of failure, reoperation and a small but not insignificant risk of not being able to walk. That can all be avoided if we just wait for things to heal.'

Mrs Stone looks out of the window at a drab townscape with silver-grey rain clouds studding the sky above, then looks back and fixes him with a stern look. 'I'd rather take the risk.'

There is an awkward silence at this stalemate.

Our boss gathers his thoughts as he plans his next move. Like all of his tribe he prides himself on his quick decision-making, and this case isn't going to plan.

He turns to me, nods and looks back at the patient with a twinkle in his eye. 'Mrs Stone, for my colleague's benefit would you kindly tell us again how you broke your hip yesterday?'

She glares at him as if to say I know what you're trying to do, then turns to me like a barrister addressing the jury. 'I have a share in a Cessna light aircraft. This morning I took off down the airfield. As you know it's been a very hot day and there was an unhelpful tailwind. When I pressed the button to retract the undercarriage it didn't seem to work. That must have provided drag and I was not clear of the tree-line as we got to the edge of the airfield. The undercarriage clipped the top of a poplar tree. Probably fifty feet off the ground, ninety knots, the plane tumbled and we crashed.

The damn undercarriage –' she shrugs, and points to her leg lying still on the bed – 'just completely stuck.'

'Thank you,' I say, suppressing my amazement that she is alive. Instead I nod my head seriously, knowing that I'm not expected to think or reply, just be a prop in Mr Maloney's rhetorical gambit.

'OK,' says Mr Maloney, 'I suppose my point is that perhaps it's time to hang up the flying goggles.'

Mrs Stone fixes him a baleful glare. 'We don't use goggles. And none of that was my fault; there was some problem with the undercarriage, I'm sure of it. Why should I be punished because of that?'

Mr Maloney agrees to get a CT scan of the hip, keep her in overnight and make a decision at the next morning's orthopaedic meeting. We gather in a cramped room with no natural light. The orthopaedic surgeons and their juniors sit in rows facing a large computer screen fixed to one wall. A couple of anaesthetists sit to one side scrutinizing their smartphones. One after the other the surgeons call out the name and date of birth of their patients, and the registrar who is piloting the computer pulls up X-rays and CT scans of the joints of that patient for discussion about the right course of action.

As each case is discussed the surgeon describes the details of the patient's story and their surgical plan. The registrar brings up images of the relevant hip, knee, foot or shoulder on to a large screen. Occasionally surgeons ask the reg to focus in on this bit of the joint at such and such an angle, and then they grill their juniors on finer anatomical and surgical points.

Some patients are decided on within a minute, some take far longer. Some patients have particularly complicated fractures or fractures around the site of a previous repair. Some patients are frail or have a medical condition that makes the anaesthetic and surgery more high risk. Some patients work in professions that rely on a certain function at that particular joint. And then there are patients of an age in whom the risks and benefits of a particular course of action are not clear-cut.

During this group analysis some in the audience are quick to comment, some hang back, some are voluble in their analysis, some more sparing. Their answers reflect their specific expertise, their level of seniority and, of course, their personality. It's clear from their comments that while all are focused on the joint shining whitely on the screen, some are less and some more interested in the person in whose body the joint resides.

Mr Maloney is pretty senior.

'Who here can fly a plane?' he asks after telling the registrar Mrs Stone's date of birth.

There's laughter around the room as they josh one of the consultants, Mr Bissett, about his three flying lessons back in the nineties.

There's a collective intake of breath when Mr Maloney explains how Mrs Stone broke her hip. The joint appears on the screen ten times life-size. Mr Maloney asks the registrar to rotate the three-dimensional image produced by the CT-scan image on the screen. It's like magic looking inside the patient's joint from every angle. You can see that there's a metal implant already in her femoral bone from a previous hip replacement, and the bone has fractured around the top of the implant, a chunk hanging slightly away from the rest of it. Her bone looks greyer than many we have seen so far today, showing how thin it is.

'I think she was lucky,' Mr Bissett says, 'just to get away with that.'

There's general agreement around the room.

'And aren't we lucky to have a resident expert on crashing aeroplanes?' Ms Nevin says.

Mr Bissett grins. 'I never crashed. Just ran out of money.'

'So here's the dilemma,' Mr Maloney says, 'give it a chance to heal by itself or go in and fix it? And if so, which method?'

It's clear after a long silence that none of the juniors seem to want to answer.

'What's her functional status?' Mr Bhatia, one of the hip specialists asks.

'She's a bit overweight, high blood pressure, otherwise no co-morbidities,' I say.

'And she wants to fly again,' Mr Maloney adds, looking at his colleagues, a half-smile on his face.

There's some laughter around the room.

'Oh dear,' says Mr Singh, the trauma specialist. 'Will she be allowed to?'

'If they find it was an equipment failure, then it will just depend on her health,' Mr Maloney says.

'I wouldn't want to fly with her,' Mr Bissett says.

'I'd rather she was flying the plane than you,' Ms Nevin says to general laughter.

'The safe thing is not to operate,' says Mr Singh. 'It may leave her with a limp, pain, and it may fracture again – only time will tell.'

'I agree with Sundeep. I'd treat it conservatively,' Mr

Walker agrees. 'We know with osteoporosis these often don't do well either way.'

'But look at the displacement,' Mr Maloney says, 'almost two centimetres.'

'Almost but not quite,' Mr Singh says. 'You're well within your rights to leave it, whereas if you operate and things go wrong, that won't look good.'

'If you're going to fix it, do it now,' says Mr Bhatia. 'She sounds like an active person, so the joint is going to get some use.' He smiles at Mr Maloney. 'Partly it depends how much of a risk she wants to take, partly it depends how careful you are of your stats.'

Mr Maloney scrutinizes the CT scan. 'John,' he says to one of the anaesthetists, 'you'd be happy for us to operate?'

'As happy as I ever am,' the anaesthetist responds. 'If she's fit enough to fly a plane, I should be able to keep her alive.'

'But is she?' Mr Smith asks, raising his hands to the heavens. 'That's the question.'

'Even with you operating, Martin, I still wouldn't want to fly with her afterwards,' Mr Bissett says.

'If you met her, you might change your mind,' Mr Maloney says.

'I got a call from a friend last night,' Mrs Stone tells us.

She is sitting in a bed up on the orthopaedic ward, a John Grisham novel lying on the pillow next to her, summer rain clattering against the windows of her hospital bay.

'He confirmed it. The tyre blew so the undercarriage couldn't retract. I knew it,' she says, passion in her eyes.

'Well, it sounds like a dangerous business either way,' Mr Maloney replies.

'No, no, it isn't. It really shouldn't be. But the heat of the day, the tailwind, the undercarriage.' She tuts and shakes her head. 'Added together it must have all been too much.'

She seems slightly unconvinced by her own analysis. 'It was a very hot day,' she repeats more firmly.

Mr Maloney looks on with his shrewd gaze. 'Now, I've discussed your case with my colleagues.'

'Good,' Mrs Stone says.

'It's a difficult call and if we operate there's a significant, maybe ten per cent chance, things will go badly wrong. Whereas if we just use a crutch and rehabilitation, we know we won't be risking further harm.'

'But that would leave an increased risk of pain, stiffness and a limp, isn't that right?' Mrs Stone counters.

'If we do the operation, the recovery period will be much longer, many months, even up to a year,' Mr Maloney says.

'But after that there's a better chance of being able to fly?' she asks.

'Well, perhaps,' Mr Maloney says. 'I'm not going to weigh in on your life and it would be up to you to decide if you wanted to try that again.'

'It's all I care about,' Mrs Stone says.

'Even after the accident?' Mr Maloney asks.

'Mr Maloney, let me explain,' she says. 'My father flew Spitfires in the war. He took me out flying when I was nine years old. I can still remember that first time. Up there in this tiny contraption, it felt like a matchbox held together with glue, millions of creatures below us and only the sun above.

'He let me use the controls when I was eleven. Oh my God. I was flying. My friends were so jealous. My mother was furious with him; she was very traditional.'

She turns away from us and looks back out at the clouds scudding through the sky, so that all we can see is her thatch of grey hair.

'When Father died I carried on.'

I look at Mr Maloney. By repute he is a very good surgeon. He is a tough boss, never shows weakness and doesn't like to see it in others.

Now Mrs Stone is looking straight at him.

'Down here my body's falling apart. I'm fat, grey, old. Up there . . .' She points out of the window at the rain-filled sky, clouds scudding past. 'Up there, when you get above the clouds, none of that matters.'

Mr Maloney smiles and nods slowly, looking Mrs Stone in the eye as he does so. 'One day someone's going to tell me I can't be a surgeon any more,' he says, 'and it's going to be hard to take, so I'll do the operation to the best of my ability, but it may not be enough.'

Mrs Stone looks at him seriously. 'Thank you.'

He pauses and looks at her to make sure she's listening. 'You'll have a long time to curse me if things go wrong.'

'I feel lucky,' Mrs Stone says.

Four Sisters

After I have shaken his small dry hand, Dmitri sits in a chair in the middle of the large Victorian consulting room, with its peeling green paint, noisy radiator and posters offering help with depression, addiction, loneliness. He is small, dapper and grey in a suit and spectacles. See Dmitri walking down the street and you'd think he was a retired solicitor or insurance clerk. You might notice a certain dignity and self-sufficiency in his face but you'd probably miss it in the few seconds before your gaze passed on to more interesting things.

'And what have you been doing today, Dmitri?' I ask.

'I've been out to the port as usual,' he says in a quiet precise voice, 'where the foot passengers come off the ferries from Scandinavia. It's cold out there today,' he says, rubbing his arms with his hands. 'There's a bitter wind.'

'Were you looking for the lady?' I ask.

'Yes,' says Dmitri, a shy smile on his face.

'And was she there?'

'No,' says Dmitri, shaking his head. 'She decided not to come.'

'How long have you been looking for her?'

He retreats back into his own thoughts. 'A long time,' he says finally.

Distantly through the high window the coffee-coloured sea boils away under a silver sky. Seagulls divebomb the water for targets under the surface that we cannot see.

'How often do you go to the port?' I ask.

'Most days,' he says.

'I know that one day she will come from Russia by boat,' he says. 'That's the way I arrived. I don't want to miss her.'

'And you're sure you'll recognize her?'

'Of course,' he says, as patiently as a teacher explaining something to a slow child.

'What does she look like?'

His face lights up. 'Oh, she's beautiful,' he says. 'She's got long blonde hair. She's tall, she's –' he pauses, as if in order to be respectful – 'beautiful. She dresses beautifully. She's very rich. Yes,' he says proudly.

'She must be sixty or seventy years old now,' I say.

'No, no,' Dmitri says. 'She is still in her twenties.'

I allow puzzlement to show on my face. Dmitri politely ignores it.

'Why did she choose you?' I ask. 'It sounds as if she could have had her pick of men?'

'She could have had anyone,' says Dmitri thoughtfully. 'Even she can't explain it. She says it was love at first sight.'

'She sounds wonderful,' I say.

'Not so wonderful as a person,' he says.

'Do you love her?'

'No,' he says. 'Not after everything she's done.'

'And what has she done?'

'She has made my life hell.'

Out on the sea a cormorant stands patiently on a buoy, wings spread to dry, as if auditioning for a coat of arms.

'What will you do if you see her?' I ask, unable to stop a frown flitting across my face. This is what Dr McCarthy has always feared, that Dmitri will actually find her.

'Tell her to leave me alone,' he says, a determined look on his face.

'Tell her?'

'Yes, tell her.'

'Do you think that will work?'

He shrugs. 'I hope so.'

'And you'd *tell* her to leave you alone, but that would be it?'

'I'm not going to hurt her,' says Dmitri, eyes glittering behind the specs. 'I'm not crazy.'

A seagull starts shrieking outside the window.

'I'm not crazy,' he says.

It seems as if Dmitri's life never really got going because of this woman. He has been partially estranged from his family, struggled to hold down and lost several jobs, he has been hospitalized several times, his marriage has been severely afflicted. And yet he remains obsessed by her.

Dr McCarthy has asked me to check in with how Dmitri is doing. I ask him if he's willing to tell me his story, and he does so happily.

Born in a village in rural Siberia, Dmitri grew up poor, helping his parents on their smallholding: a grove of larch trees, sheep and a few pigs. In his late teens he had planned to move to the regional city for work but then he was chosen by a woman, who he always refers to abstractly as 'the *devushka*' or 'lady' and it never happened.

Dmitri had never met the lady but he knew exactly what she looked like. She lived in a big house not too far from his village. She was rich and beautiful, her blondness a rarity in his part of the Soviet Union. For reasons that were still mysterious to Dmitri she chose him as her beau.

Although her attention flattered him, from the beginning of their relationship the lady was domineering and cruel, putting him down whenever she got the chance, making him question his abilities, question his actions, question his manhood. This, he thinks, was why he never made it to the city. It's not clear if he had some sort of breakdown at this point but a few years later he was together enough to emigrate to England, arriving by ship from a northern Soviet port. He can't remember if he was trying to escape the lady, but it didn't work that way.

It turned out the lady was so rich that she had elaborate technological means of observing Dmitri even from a distance of four thousand miles. She had some sort of computerized studio from which she could monitor his movements, actions, words and even his thoughts. She was also able to use the technology to communicate her thoughts to him directly, something she was doing constantly. Dmitri wasn't really able to explain it – well, why should he be able to? After all, the lady didn't want him to understand. What he was quite aware of was that she felt rejected by his travelling overseas, and her thoughts were mostly critical and abusive.

Dmitri found work in the port town he arrived in and settled there, the lady never far from his thoughts. Several years later, he met a local woman named Mary at a dance, and married her.

The lady was furious, ridiculed Mary and warned Dmitri against the union. The lady was in love with him; she had chosen him, she was rich and powerful and she was horrified to be cast over. Every day she told Dmitri that Mary was ugly, poor and worthless, and that there was no love in the marriage. Her efforts sometimes extended to controlling his thoughts, his words and his body. Sometimes she made him cold or unfriendly to his wife. Occasionally she goaded him into saying sharp or hurtful things to her.

Being caught between the lady and his wife was unimaginably stressful for Dmitri and eventually, in his late twenties, he had some sort of breakdown and was hospitalized. He was diagnosed with paranoid schizophrenia and put on monthly injections of antipsychotic medication. He left hospital after several months and has been getting these injections and seeing psychiatrists ever since.

After his hospitalization Dmitri stayed at home for a while, just sleeping and sitting out in a chair, scarcely eating or talking, unable to work and totally reliant on his wife. During this period the lady lambasted him for his weakness, for his failure as a breadwinner, for bringing shame to his parents, for his lack of virility with Mary. At this time Dmitri wondered if he would ever get his life back on track.

He pauses for a moment in his story. He looks haunted by these memories. He looks small here in the middle of the vast clinic room, in the middle of the city.

'That's when the engineer came along,' Dmitri says. 'She helped me get back on my feet.'

'Which engineer is that?' I ask.

'The lady's sister,' says Dmitri with a wry smile. 'She's an engineer from back home in Siberia. She defends me from the lady. Fortunately she is a very smart woman. Smart in intelligence and in dress. She always wears a good dress, an expensive watch, has a good haircut.'

Dmitri breaks off, a look of gratitude on his face. 'Really, without her I don't know if I could have survived all these years. She knows how the world works. She protects me from the lady.'

'How does she do that?' I ask.

'Oh, she has her ways. She reasons with the lady, argues with her, advises me on what to do and what not to do. She is very clever. And she understands the way the lady's mind works because they grew up together. Back then, shortly after my breakdown, she convinced the lady that I could work again. It was like I was under some sort of curse, but the engineer convinced her to lift it.'

Dmitri managed to get a job as a porter in one of the city's grander hotels, a place where he worked for the next fifteen years. He enjoyed his work, the insight he had into the daily lives of others, meeting important people, becoming part of the family of the hotel. But during this time there were still tortuous negotiations and schemes between the lady, persecuting him, and the engineer, defending him, with Dmitri a pawn in their byzantine game. For some time he became quite ill again, and sometimes he had to take sick leave or increase his medications.

'Why did the engineer come to help you?' I ask.

He smiles shyly again. 'I don't understand it. I suppose as I have been cursed with the lady so I've been blessed with the engineer.'

'How does she communicate with you?'

'She speaks to me directly. I cannot see her, but she talks to me.'

'Can you hear her now?'

'Not at the moment. But she's listening to our conversation. She approves of me talking to you.'

A seagull shrieks outside the window, and Dmitri sits

there, so far away from me across the room that he looks as much a spectator as a participant in his story.

'I don't know if I would have survived this long without the engineer, or without Doctor McCarthy.'

It was during Dmitri's time working at the hotel that Dr McCarthy became his psychiatrist and he has been seeing him regularly ever since.

'You get on well with him?'

'He listens to me and he understands me; that is very important for a man in my position,' he says.

Over the years Dmitri's illness has waxed and waned, but for decades he managed to keep his job at the hotel and suppress his inner life so that those around him were scarcely aware of it. His sometimes eccentric behaviour was tolerated. Then at one point Dmitri's boss became concerned when he saw Dmitri in the vacant ballroom gesticulating and commanding the empty air to go away. The hotel asked for input from Dr McCarthy and after a correspondence they agreed to keep Dmitri on. But by this time he felt the strain of keeping the lady hidden from the customers and colleagues had become too great, and he resigned.

Around the time he stopped working the lady's youngest two sisters – one a dentist, one a teacher – gained access to the computer room in Siberia. They were jealous of the lady, he explains. Like her they were both deeply attracted to Dmitri and wanted him for themselves. They would bicker among themselves as to who should have him, who was most worthy of him. The engineer tried to intercede and smooth things out between them but they would accuse the engineer of wanting Dmitri for herself. When the teacher or dentist got the upper hand the lady would cause Dmitri all sorts of problems and the engineer would have to defend him from her scorn and jealousy. When the lady was back on top Dmitri would be aware of a concerted campaign of the teacher and dentist against their older sister.

'And what do they want from you?'

'I think they want me as a sort of trophy,' he says, 'to be theirs to be able to show off about me.'

His modest smile broadens; he looks pleased with himself. 'Yes. They argue among each other. They make my life a misery with their attention.

'They're a very, very beautiful family. Four beautiful sisters. I think the teacher is the most beautiful.' Suddenly Dmitri looks troubled. 'No,' he says. 'No.'

He stares across the room intently as if listening to someone else. After a minute his face relaxes and he looks at me. 'The lady doesn't agree.' He smiles shyly again. 'She's always been so jealous of my attention.'

I look at Dmitri, a small innocuous-looking man with this baroque cast of characters in his head.

'What's her name?' I ask.

'Whose?'

'The lady's.'

'I don't know,' he says.

'The engineer's? The teacher's? The dentist's?'

'I don't know.'

'You don't know?'

'The names don't matter,' he says quietly.

Dmitri has not worked since leaving his job at the hotel two decades ago. He reads books, watches TV, listens to and deals with the cacophony in his head. He spends five mornings a week going to the ferry port, hoping to see the lady.

'Are you still married?' I ask.

'Yes,' he says. 'I'm still married to Mary. She has stuck with me.' He looks out of the window at the sea. 'We no longer dance.' A half-smile materializes on his face. 'She's annoyed that I go to the port; she nags me to get a hobby, to do something else with my time.'

'But you still go.'

'It's my life,' Dmitri says.

'Do you have children?'

'Mary wanted children. But we couldn't have any. The lady wouldn't allow it.'

'How did she stop you having children?'

'Well, she would block us. You know . . .' He looks at me awkwardly. 'In bed.'

'OK,' I say.

'She still blocks me,' Dmitri continues, talking so quietly he's almost talking to himself. 'I cannot embrace my wife.'

'Did you want children?' I ask.

A look of pain flashes across his face, then disappears. 'It would have made my wife happy,' he says, 'and I owe her a lot.'

I think about his wife, a flesh and blood woman, who has spent decades living alongside an invisible enemy who has stolen so much from her.

'What does Mary think of all this?'

'She is very understanding. She used to come with me to these appointments, but . . .' He pauses and swallows back emotion, then tries to set his face. 'She doesn't come any more; she says she finds it too sad.'

*

We sit in silence, Dmitri staring out of the window. I look at this gentle dapper man carrying an illness known more for its loud outbursts than its quiet inexorable sapping of life and opportunity, the way it stains everything with its own false meaning. Have these delusions been a curse, a form of protection or both? How far has the boy from Siberia really travelled? Walking down to the port where he arrived in England forty-five years ago to look for this fantasy, this spectre, perhaps almost hoping to meet his younger self coming off the ship.

Outside the sun makes a brief appearance out from behind the thick clouds and the sea is dazzling with light. I am professionally obliged to ask the next question but it makes me feel awkward given the centrality of his delusions.

'Do you think the lady is part of the illness? Part of the schizophrenia?'

He looks at me with curiosity and thinks for a long time. 'She helped cause the illness,' he says, 'but she's real.'

'Real as in a real person?'

He looks at me quizzically. 'Yes, a real person.'

It feels disrespectful but I persevere. 'Sitting in a room somewhere in Russia at her computer?'

'Yes, all of these things.'

'Do you understand that for someone like me to hear that a real woman is sitting somewhere contacting and controlling you through some amazing technology all sounds very unlikely? It seems to me the lady and the sisters are all part of the illness.'

Dmitri looks patiently at me, the schoolteacher with his slightly dim pupil. 'Of course I understand that. People have been telling me that for years. You're not supposed to understand. She manages it that way. She's a lot more power-ful than you doctors.'

He lapses into silence, staring hard at the floor. He suddenly looks exhausted.

We sit there for a while in the consultation room. Through the high window the wind has whipped up rollers on the surface of the sea, confronting the city with an inverted world where almost everything happens beneath and out of sight.

'It seems to me the lady is the defining feature of your life.'

At this Dmitri looks thoughtful. 'Perhaps you're right,' he says, and then fixes me in his gaze. 'She knows me better than anyone else,' he says simply, 'and she chose me.'

'And tell me again why you are going to the ferry port?'

Dmitri turns and looks out of the window towards the brown seething sea.

'I want to meet her,' he says.

Stroke

The elderly woman in the spartan A & E cubicle is wearing a thick string of pearls and a tweed suit. She has a plump, ruddy, asymmetrical face. One half of it slumps downwards like a basset hound's while the other remains aloft. When she smiles only the high side rises, making her mouth a sideways 'S'.

I ask her to raise her eyebrows. Fluffy and white they both shoot up towards her hairline in a vaguely comical fashion, crinkling her brow. This means she's had a stroke, not a facial palsy, and time is of the essence.

'When did your face start drooping?' I ask.

If the answer is a time in the last four and a half hours, we will need an immediate CT scan of her head, and if that shows a blood clot in the brain, we will quickly give her a drug to try to melt the clot and reverse her symptoms. If, on the other hand, it has been four hours and thirty-one minutes or longer since the symptoms started, we will simply have to see what sort of recovery nature holds in store.

'Oh, Charles,' she says in a plummy voice, slightly slurring because of the partial paralysis of her face, 'when did I first start looking like this horror?'

An elderly man in a tweed suit perching politely on the edge of a chair at the foot of the bed ponders this. He has a silk cravat round his neck, patent-leather shoes flat on the floor, hands resting on a walking stick, back ramrod straight.

'Oh, I don't know, Cecily. Now, let me think, when was it? Perhaps the sole.'

'No, no, Charles. I couldn't manage the sole, which was a great shame,' she says, fixing me a gaze, 'because it looked lovely.'

'It doesn't have to be that precise,' I say, 'just roughly. Was it after midday or before?'

'Of course, doctor,' she says obediently, 'of course.'

She frowns and again I am transfixed by her fluffy eyebrows, which are functioning normally, a reminder that we must get on with it.

'Before or after midday,' I say, prompting her.

Then her face lights up. 'I think it was the soup when I began to have the trouble.'

The elderly man's face lights up. 'That's it,' he says, 'the soup; it began to dribble out of the side of your mouth. I felt sorry for you because it was very nice. And I remember your napkin was covered.'

'Please, Charles,' she admonishes her husband, 'don't distress this young man.'

'What time did you eat the soup?' I ask.

'Well, we have lunch at one o'clock sharp, so it would have been about one,' the man says. 'Isn't that right, Cecily?'

'Like clockwork,' she says.

I look at my watch; it's two minutes to five. If we can get her into the scanner sharpish, there should still be time to bust the clot.

'And that's when the symptoms started?' I ask. 'During the soup, not earlier?'

'During the soup,' Cecily confirms.

'Well, that's four hours ago,' I say, 'so we will need to

quickly scan your head and may be able to give a medicine to
try to melt the clot.'

'Hmmm,' says Charles.

'What is it?' I ask.

'I'm afraid I don't quite agree with your arithmetic.'

'How come?'

'It's rather more than four hours,' he says.

'I think,' says Cecily, 'you thought we meant luncheon
today.'

Charles laughs. 'Oh, I see. Yes. But we eat fish on
Fridays.'

'Friday?' I say. 'This happened during the soup you ate at
lunch *yesterday*?'

'Before the fish,' Charles says.

'So, to be clear, it's Saturday today.'

'Of course it is,' she says. 'We've just had the nephews and
nieces round for tea.'

'And it was *yesterday* when your face started drooping,' I
say, not wanting to consign Cecily to a lifetime of disability
because of a misunderstanding over the day of the week
when fish is best eaten.

The patient nods firmly.

'During the soup,' Charles adds.

'And it's been like this ever since?' I ask.

'Yes,' she says, picking up on my incredulity.

'OK,' I say, thinking, the damage is done, there's no need
to rush.

'OK,' I repeat, trying to slow my thoughts down, to quell
my frustration.

I ask Cecily some background questions to assess the
things that made her more at risk of a stroke, things we might

be able to change to make it less likely to happen again: other diseases, family history of such diseases and some lifestyle questions.

'Do you smoke?'

'Just the occasional cigarette now,' she says.

'And alcohol?'

'Oh, yes please,' she says loudly, amused at her own joke.

I can't help myself laughing.

'Now, now, Cecily,' Charles says from behind me. 'Try to behave.'

Now I feel able to come back to the question that has been burning me.

'Can I ask why you left it so long to come here?'

'Oh,' Cecily says, 'it seemed like such a minor thing. It wasn't painful and it didn't seem life-threatening. And we know how busy you are here. It was only our niece who saw us today and bullied us into calling the ambulance. Ridiculous really, we could have driven.'

My mind returns to all the people I've seen in this department who didn't need to come. I remember a few months back Kevin and his insects and his symptom-free allergic reactions.

'I did tell you, Cecily,' her husband says, picking up on the hint of admonition in my tone, 'but you wouldn't hear any of it.'

'That's true, Charles,' says Cecily. 'I thought you were making a fuss. And I suppose I don't like hospitals.'

Charles raises bushy grey eyebrows as he speaks directly to me. 'She won't mind me telling you, doctor, she's always been the stubborn sort.'

'Often an admirable quality,' I say. I approach the bed. 'Do you know what's happened to you, Cecily?'

She looks at me with serious pale blue eyes from her lop-sided face. 'Have I had a small stroke?'

'You have indeed,' I say. 'We can give medicine to try to stop it from happening again and we'll get you doing exercises with our team to help try to reduce the drooping and improve your speech, but there are no guarantees that your face will regain its former function.'

'I understand,' she says.

'If anything like this ever happens again,' I say, 'I want you to know that we come to work here precisely to help people like you. We want you to call the ambulance immediately, because if you come here quickly there's a better chance of us fixing things. Please tell me you will.'

Cecily frowns. 'Yes, doctor, I will.'

'Thank you,' I say.

'I'll hold you to that, young Cecily,' her husband says. 'I don't much fancy the idea of being stuck down here without you.'

Later I come in to say we have a bed arranged on the stroke ward.

Cecily is standing in front of the small mirror in the cubicle pulling the slouching side of her face up to make it symmetrical. Charles stands dutifully behind her looking at her reflection.

'It's not such a big thing,' she says half to herself. 'The dogs won't care how I look anyway.'

Charles places a hand on her tweedy shoulder. 'You're still beautiful, darling.'

She bends an arm and places her hand on top of his. She closes her eyes and half her face smiles.

The Fall

Nancy is tall, with a shock of red hair, and a spherical body on stick-thin legs that makes every doctor who meets her think she has an undiagnosed pituitary problem. She hasn't but she has a lot of others.

'When I die I'm going to leave my brain to medical science,' Nancy likes to tell me, 'and my body to McDonald's.'

'Sounds the right way round,' I say.

She is pleased by the implied rudeness.

'Did you come up with that line?' I ask.

'I'm not sure if I made it up or stole it,' Nancy says. 'The universal consciousness is so strong these days.'

I laugh out loud.

'I'm not sure McDonald's would take me,' she adds mournfully, pointing at her large torso.

She sits in the middle of her new flat, boxes still stacked against one wall; a fake vintage wooden sign propped up against them. It says HOME SWEET HOME. A livid purple bruise covers one half of her face. She is talking in that slow, slurred, careful voice of hers, the received pronunciation of her socially privileged upbringing shining through the dilapidation of the last sixty years. Her involuntary lip-smacking reveals a single tooth that points to the heavens, the result of decades of antipsychotic medication and poor nutrition.

As far back as our medical records go they show that she has suffered mental ill health, been in and out of hospital and medicated to the hilt. She is now on nine regular medications a day to manage her mood, her mind, her pain and the physical ailments she has picked up over the years. Senior doctors at the practice tell me she is much more stable, much calmer than she ever used to be, and it's true I've never known her to be angry or upset. She is always lucid, funny and disgruntled.

Now she has started falling. It has happened three times in the last month, and this last time she hurt herself so badly she had to be in hospital for twenty-four hours for them to rule out fractures and check there wasn't a new illness causing her to fall. But their conclusion is the same as mine: that a combination of weak limbs, excess body weight and the side effects of her medication are the problem. Nothing easy to fix. I explain this and my plan to arrange for her to have some physiotherapy and to reduce some of her medication doses.

Nancy's mouth curls into an impish grin and a glint alights in her eyes. 'I know the letter said I fell, Doctor Tem-ple-ton,' she says, 'but between you and me I did this to myself.' She points at her bulging bruised right eye socket. 'I threw myself at the door in frus-tration. Then when I saw how badly I was hurt I called the paramedics.' She can see me frown. 'I know that was naughty of me.'

'What was the frustration about?'

'This,' she says, looking around. 'This place.'

'But this is what you wanted,' I say. 'This is what all those people spent the last year fighting to get you.'

'I know, and I'm appreciative,' she says, 'but I don't like it.'

'But this is better, isn't it? This is a nice flat. It's clean, light, and you've got a lovely view out the window there of that park . . .'

'You sound like an estate agent.'

'You have the carers right here to look after you if you need them.'

'I don't like them looking in on me,' she says. 'I want my own privacy.'

'But you need them,' I say. 'You don't really have an option, Nancy.'

'But I can't get out like I want to,' she says, 'because of the pain in my legs.'

'And you couldn't get out of the last place because of the stairs,' I say. 'At least there's a lift here so you can be wheeled if you want.'

'But there's no one around to wheel me,' she says, 'and once I'm out where would I go?'

I hold out my arms as if to say what can we do about it? What can we do about the body that is too large for your legs to support yourself in walking more than a few metres? What can we do about your loneliness when you refuse to attend the groups and social events on offer? What can we do about the deprivations and lunacies of the past?

'I know,' she says, as if understanding everything unsaid. 'I know. I'm just telling you.'

'It's not sensible to throw yourself around,' I say. 'You could really hurt yourself.'

'I know,' she says again.

'What can I do to help, Nancy?' I ask.

'Just stay here a while,' she says.

Nancy is in a reflective mood and she tells me a story from her childhood about seeing her father, who was a lawyer, beating their dog and how she never stopped hating him from then on.

'Daddy never touched me but he was such an angry man. I was always scared of him. When I was a teenager I would fly into rages myself and I hated it. I didn't want to be like him but I couldn't control it.'

Nancy described her mother as a prim, snooty individual, always critical of the way other people dressed or spoke or lived. 'Mummy was thick as two short planks. She was so stiff you'd have to saw her up and set her on fire to get any warmth from her.'

Nancy had mammoth temper tantrums as a young child where she would throw herself on the floor for half an hour at a time. She was manifestly troubled by the time she started school.

'My parents said I'd always been a problem child. I suppose they didn't know anything about children's brains in those days,' she said. 'There was a lot of stigma attached, so my mum didn't want to face it.'

Her brother was packed off to boarding school from a young age and she had no allies at home. One evening, aged fifteen, she smashed up her mum's favourite Royal Doulton ornaments. That night she was taken in for the first of many inpatient stays on a mental health ward. Nancy saw this as a sort of punishment by her parents.

'Just the kind of tit for tat Mummy would employ. A month in the loony bin to pay for her china,' she says to me bitterly all these years later. She describes an adulthood in which she was never long enough out of the 'bin' to 'ever really get going'.

'They could never seem to quite work out what I have. They changed their minds all the time. I suppose it doesn't really matter now. I couldn't wait to get away from my parents, but the more unwell I got, the harder it became.'

She never managed to work and has spent a life navigating benefits. She has never had an intimate relationship and has alienated most of the friends and family she had. When her parents died she hadn't seen either of them for years. The only human contact she has now is carers, the mental health nurse and us at the surgery.

Hearing her run through it all I realize how each new setback added to an already insurmountable set of challenges. She really never did get going. And she's blunt enough in her recollection to reveal the threads of self-destruction woven through her life. Whenever things seemed to be improving she would do something crazy. Unique among all the animals, I think, is the human ability for self-sabotage.

'I've been my own worst enemy, haven't I?' she says, regretful, but pleased to have an audience.

'It's never too late to change,' I say, doubting my own words.

'I think maybe the best place for me is hospital,' she says. 'At least there I get three square meals and some company.'

'Hospital is not a sensible place for you,' I say.

'Don't believe everything you hear,' she says. 'The company's lousy but the food's good.'

'You need to get these boxes unpacked,' I say, 'then we need to do something about your loneliness.'

'You come and visit me,' she says slyly.

'That's not a long-term solution,' I reply.

As we are talking the first cases of a new infectious disease are spreading among people in China and soon enough we are caught up in the first wave of this disease. We begin to do most of our consultations via phone and video and I call

Nancy one day to check how she is doing, but there is no answer and I leave a message.

A few days later I get a hospital letter stating that she has had another fall and was admitted and needed three days on a ward to get her pain under control. I wonder about the word 'fall' given that, again, the hospital have found nothing new wrong with Nancy and given her propensity for throwing herself around. Indeed the letter mentions that she was not keen to leave and they sound quite stressed about how difficult it was to convince her to go. They also add that she looks as if she has a pituitary problem.

'Did you really fall, Nancy?' I ask when I get her on the phone.

'Cross my heart and hope to die, Doctor Templeton. I tripped over my walking frame.' She chuckles.

'Really, Nancy?'

There is a long pause.

'Well, I don't quite remember what happened,' she says. There is another pause. 'I know I felt dreadfully frustrated just beforehand. Perhaps I did do it on purpose.'

'Nancy,' I say, 'this is not on.'

'I know,' she says, and sounds more remorseful than I expected.

'They weren't quite as friendly as usual,' she says. 'They were worried about this coronavirus thingy.'

'They have a lot on their plate,' I say. 'They don't need any unnecessary work.'

'But it's this damn pain in my legs, Doctor Templeton.'

'And we've already got you on every painkiller known to humanity,' I say.

'I know,' she says. 'I'm rattling with all those pills.'

'You are. And there's nothing different they can do in hospital.'

'I know,' she says again, 'but it's still damn painful. And sleep . . . it's so hard to get to sleep.'

'I'll try to think of something,' I say for want of anything better.

'Come and visit,' she says.

'Visiting's out now unless absolutely necessary,' I say.

'Bloody pandemic,' she says.

A few days later I ring Nancy to check how she's getting on at home but there is no answer and I leave a message. A few days after that I get another hospital letter. The day after I had spoken to her Nancy had fallen again it explains. This time it seemed to have been a genuine fall. On arrival at the hospital she had been found to have a raging lung infection and her oxygen levels were precarious. They had diagnosed Covid-19 through a CT scan. (The way the timings worked she must have picked it up on her previous self-generated hospital visit, I think to myself.) Nancy's condition had deteriorated rapidly and, given her physical frailty, she was not considered a candidate for ventilation and intensive care. A day after arriving at hospital, Nancy had died.

The news hits me like a punch in the stomach. I liked Nancy. She had a lot of problems. And none of them seemed like they would get anything but worse. But she had a glint in her eye and tremendous endurance and spirit.

I worry I did something or failed to do something that contributed to her death, that I wasn't tough enough with her or convincing enough about the risks of harming herself.

Later on, perhaps trying to make myself feel better, I imagine the progress of the virus and Nancy as they made their way towards their fateful meeting as being inevitable. The virus falling in droplets from bat to bat to bat to pangolin to human to human to human, falling and falling and falling as it travelled around the world. And Nancy, who had been falling to the floor since she was two years old and had been falling in and out of hospital ever since, falling in one time too many.

Either way Nancy was lonely and wanted to be in hospital. And the virus, which trails a pandemic of loneliness in its wake but is always keen to meet new people, was waiting there with open arms.

Bob

One day on the morning ward round we are surprised to find that Janet has turned into a man.

When we left the previous evening she lay propped up in the bed in Side Room 7 recovering from a fractured hip, lucid as glass, talking about a great-niece who paints surrealist portraits in Canada with her loud West Country voice, frizzy grey hair and impressive stubble.

This morning the room looks the same: the small fake wooden cabinet with black slippers in front; the view of the car park fringed by the plastic spikes to keep the pigeons from roosting; the faded print on the wall of a Provençal river at night. But instead of Janet there is a man lying on the bed, dozing in the faint winter light.

His head looks large in comparison to the stick-like limbs that emerge from the pale green hospital-issue pyjamas. He has milky skin and a large upper lip with a prominent philtrum coated with a dark moustache.

There is some muttering among the junior doctors and nurses. Our primary job is to know the patients, and no one knows anything about this one, let alone what the hell has happened to Janet.

Our consultant gently shakes the man by the shoulder. The man inhales one last contented sleeping breath then opens his eyes and enters our world.

'Oo, wha, huh,' he says, blinking at the crowd of people gathered around him.

'Hello?' says the consultant politely.

''Ello,' says the man warily.

'Sorry to wake you. My name is Doctor Esfahani.'

'Uhh,' says the man, shaking his head, as if to rattle the sleep out. 'I'm Bob. Ooh are you?'

'Doctor Esfahani,' he says a bit louder.

'No need to shout,' says Bob. 'My 'earing's fine.' He holds out a hand that Dr Esfahani takes.

'What'd you say yer name was?' Bob says, looking confused, lying in bed drenched in sunshine, surrounded by strangers.

'Doctor Esfahani. You're in hospital,' says Dr Esfahani.

'Why?' asks Bob.

Dr Esfahani smiles and looks embarrassed. 'I don't know,' he says. 'We're just trying to find out.'

We stand in awkward silence. Rashmi enters the room wearing baggy blue scrubs, looking flustered, eyes drawn, the wrong side of a night shift spent running around the whole hospital.

Dr Esfahani excuses himself to Bob and we shuffle outside to talk to her.

'Sorry, Doctor Esfahani, I got caught up in handover.'

'No problem.'

'Just to let you know, Janet died last night. I've no idea why. I wasn't even called by the nurses until after she'd gone.'

There's muttering among our crew. Janet dead?

She seemed well yesterday, I think.

Dr Esfahani absorbs the information calmly and no doubt

mentally files finding out what happened with Janet on to his to-do list for after the ward round.

'Bob in here –' he points over his shoulder – 'was just asking why he's in hospital. I said I didn't know.'

Rashmi rifles through her clipboard of lists. 'Bob . . . Bob . . . Bob . . .' She shakes her head.

Someone standing next to her points to *Robert S, Side Room 7.*

'Oh, yes,' she says. It's clear from her baffled air that she knows nothing about it. 'It just says dementia. Not really sure why he's in – maybe a social?'

We return to the room to talk to Bob.

''Ow you all doing?' he asks, looking unhappy under the framed print of a blue river in a blue night with its golden spiral stars and leaking house lights. 'I'm Bob. Ooh are you?'

The last thing you need if you have dementia is to wake up in a strange place and start getting the third degree by a group of strangers.

Dr Esfahani introduces himself again, and the rest of us throw him a few nods and half-smiles.

'So how are you feeling, Bob?' asks Dr Esfahani.

'Good,' he says.

'How are things at home?'

'Good,' Bob says.

'Who do you live with?'

'I'm on me own,' he says.

'Are you managing OK?'

Bob looks at Dr Esfahani suspiciously and folds his arms. 'Very well, thank you.'

A pigeon has landed and is sitting awkwardly on the window-sill stuck between two plastic spikes, cooing.

Dr Esfahani does a cursory physical examination. When he has finished he thanks Bob for his time, saying someone will come back later to discuss things.

'When can I go home?' asks Bob, completely baffled.

Dr Esfahani smiles ruefully. 'We need to find out why you're here first.'

When the ward sister gets out of her meeting she explains that Rashmi's guess was right. Bob is here 'on a social'. Living alone in a small terraced house in town he has been getting gradually more demented over the last year. His closest family member is a niece with young kids of her own, unable to take him in to her tiny flat. Bob is unwilling to move to a nursing home and unable to afford to. He isn't poor enough to qualify for a state-funded place, but his only money is tied up in his house. As the dementia has progressed his driving licence and car have been removed and he has exploded his microwave oven. His niece has become increasingly concerned about his house and his safety. Bob has been too proud or confused to let carers come in. Then yesterday Bob fell and wasn't able to get off the floor. The paramedics brought him to hospital. But the tests haven't shown anything wrong with him bar the dementia and a general frailty and now the hospital are stuck with him. We can't send him home as it's unsafe. It's winter and there are no beds available in the hospital-affiliated nursing homes. But until someone – Bob, the local council or the NHS – stumps up for a regular nursing home place he remains our patient, taking up a valuable and costly winter bed to no real purpose.

*

When I go to tell Bob the news I find him sporting a pair of large squarish black-framed specs and reading a newspaper.

I perch on the side of the bed and explain that we want him to stay until we get the home situation sorted out.

'So you're sayin' that I'm well,' says Bob.

'Yes . . . apart from the dementia,' I say.

'I'm well, but I 'ave to stay in hospital.' He shakes his head. 'You're crackers,' he says, laying the newspaper down on the bed, which I notice he was reading upside down. 'I thought you lads were stuffed to the gills?'

'It's pretty busy,' I say, 'but . . . we don't think your home environment is safe.'

'So I can't go home?' Bob clarifies.

I pause. In theory he can do what he wants but in practice this is catch-22 territory. We will allow him to make the decision to stay, but if he chooses to leave we will hold him on the grounds of an inability to make rational decisions, even though the desire to leave is pretty rational. We don't really want him here and he doesn't want to be here, but nonetheless he must stay.

'We'd rather you agree to stay in hospital,' I say. 'The food's not bad, I'm told.'

He looks me up and down. 'You remind me of someone,' he says. 'Can't remember 'oo.'

I laugh. 'Just give us some time to make sure we can keep you safe,' I say.

He holds out a hand to shake mine as if we're concluding a business deal. 'All right, I'll stay,' he says.

On the next morning's ward round we find Bob has been moved to a four-bedded bay in the main area of the ward. A move made out of necessity as the side room was needed for a dying patient, but almost guaranteed to confuse someone like Bob with dementia.

All the patients are in nightwear; all the staff in daywear. We're with another long-term patient in the same bay and my concentration is lagging as Dr Esfahani talks to him when I notice Bob is chuckling to himself. He's sitting out in the chair next to his bed in pale green pyjamas and a faded brown paisley dressing gown.

Bob has a twinkle in his eye. I see that he's looking past the central nurse's station to the other bay where Sally, one of the nurses, is making a bed. Bob chuckles again, then tuts.

'Look at 'im,' he says loudly to nobody in particular, waving an arm in the direction of Sally.

'Oh dear, oh dear,' he says, shaking his head. ''E's doing it all wrong.' Then he projects his voice, confidently declaiming across the crowded ward, 'You can't do it like that. Yer can't knead the dough that way; it'll never rise.'

Phil, the patient in the neighbouring bed, looks riled. Phil has a bald dome fringed with curls, wire specs on. He's a scarecrow figure with a purple-and-white-striped towelling gown and a purple nose. He looks like a mad professor.

'Oh gawd, show 'em 'ow it's done, Douglas,' bellows Bob straight past Phil. 'We'll never get this order out at this rate.' Then he starts chuckling to himself. 'Jesus! If my brother catches 'im doin' it like that there'll be hell to pay.'

'Excuse me,' says Phil loudly. He is usually quiet and retiring but has a bladder infection that has made him irritable and Bob's hollering is winding him up. 'Pipe down, will you?'

'You leave it alone, sunshine,' says Bob. 'I'm just trying to help.'

'Just cork it,' Phil says angrily, shaking a fist in Bob's direction.

'You've never dealt with the loaves,' says Bob, incredulous at Phil's insubordination. 'You stick to your order book.'

'I'll tell you where you can stick your order book,' says Phil, clearly annoyed by Bob's attitude. 'Don't you tell me what to do, you bastard.'

I move across. 'Gents, can we settle down a bit, please? You're on a hospital ward. There are sick people here.'

Phil subsides back to his usual quiet self, muttering, but Bob looks crestfallen.

Hospital? Ill? He was a man in his prime, lording it about in his place of work. I feel guilty for bringing him crashing down to earth.

Over the short winter days and long winter nights that gently extend into weeks Bob becomes the emotional fulcrum of the ward. When he's jovial the place is fun, when he's subdued things are calm and when he's riled the ward gets fiery. We never know what we're going to get. Some days he is more lucid than others; other days he swings from clarity to confusion several times.

He generally seems happier when he is occupying some area of his past. When he mistakes the ward for the large bakery firm where he worked for forty years he resumes his role as deputy manager with aplomb. When the volunteers come in and arrange a tea dance for the patients he happily returns to the post-Second World War world of 'The White Cliffs of Dover'. When he imagines himself down the pub with the nurse as his drinking buddy, he's in his element. But when reality intrudes, or when he is caught on the rim between the past and the present, things get difficult.

When Olive, the ward Labrador, is brought in to cheer up the patients he recognizes her as Lofty, his brother's dog. This pleases him no end, until he begins to wonder where his brother is, and it dawns on him that things aren't quite as he's seeing them, and he gets frightened and starts raging.

And when Bob – caught up in the world of memory back when he was in control of his own life, could do what he wanted, could go where he pleased – tries to leave the ward, our trump card is to burst the bubble and remind him where he is and when it is. This always feels like a deep betrayal.

Because these attempts at escape happen so often we get a psychiatrist to come in and do a so-called Deprivation of Liberty order so we're covered legally. The psychiatrist is a patronizing man sporting a bow tie and a shaven head, and seems annoyed at having to do this menial and time-consuming task.

'How hard have you looked for alternative aetiologies?' he asks us junior doctors sternly. 'Other organic problems? Have you even bothered to do a CT head?'

I point out that Bob was diagnosed with dementia a year ago in memory clinic and there is no sign of any delirium or anything that might cause additionally erratic behaviour.

'Hmmmm, so you haven't bothered, is that right?' the psychiatrist says.

Bob is irritated by his manner and speaks directly to the psychiatrist. 'Are you bothering Douglas?' he asks.

The psychiatrist ignores him. 'Please arrange a CT scan of his head immediately and I'll come back when it's done.'

Bob explodes at him. 'If you had anything in your head apart from shit, you'd know better than to talk to Douglas like that.'

The psychiatrist huffs and puffs. 'Excuse me, Mister, erm, Mister . . .'

'It won't end well for you, sunshine,' Bob says, shaking a fist from his chair.

I leave them to it.

It takes a week to get the CT scan, which shows, as expected, the accelerated brain shrinkage of dementia and for the psychiatrist to return and sign the form. Several weeks later Steve, a laddish physiotherapist sporting a white polo shirt and a goatee beard, comes on to the ward to try to get Bob doing some exercises. We know inactivity for someone Bob's age leads to loss of muscle and bone density that can take months of activity to recover, one of many reasons why hospital stays for the elderly can be fatal.

Bob is sitting in his chair mulling something over and Steve breaks his reverie. 'Hey, Bob,' he says with a light Aussie drawl, 'I've been asked to get you to work on your quads.'

Bob looks Steve up and down and curls his long upper lip and moustache. 'I'm not interested,' he says. 'Never 'ave been, never will.'

'I'll just show you a few leg exercises,' says Steve. 'They'll help keep your strength up.'

'There's no point,' Bob says, 'I'm not interested.'

Steve chuckles. 'If I can just show you a few exercises, Bob, then I'll get out of your hair.'

'Yer wasting yer time,' Bob says, needle entering his voice. 'I'll never vote for you. None of us ever did.'

'I'm not asking you to vote for me, Bob, just learn a few exercises; it won't take long,' Steve wheedles.

Bob explodes with rage. 'I've told you I'm not interested, you smarmy bastard,' he shouts. 'Your lot 'ave torn this country a new arsehole and dropped three massive turds ert of it: Thatcher, Major and whatshisname.'

Steve backs away. 'Listen, Bob, why don't I come back later to see if you change your mind?'

'Never,' shouts Bob. 'I'll never change my mind.'

'Oh, do shut up,' says Phil, shaking his fist from his chair a bed's width away.

'What do you know,' shouts Bob, 'you loony?'

'A lot more than you, you bastard,' Phil retorts. 'If your lot were running the place, we'd all be picking through the rubbish bins for our food.'

'You never let it rest, do you?' says Bob, shaking his head. 'I'd rather pick my own scraps than have them dropping from your filthy table.'

'Oh, you would, would you?' says Phil, glowering. 'At least we have a table, not eating from the floor.'

'I'll show you the floor,' says Bob. He begins to raise his scrawny frame from his chair, finally doing the very thing Steve wanted him to.

I get up from where I'm sitting writing notes. 'Bob, can I help you?' I ask, standing a few metres back from him as he tries to stagger up.

'I can 'andle this meself,' he says, getting unsteadily to his feet.

Reluctantly I pull the situational trick. 'You're in hospital, you know?' I say. 'It's the year two thousand and—.'

'Get out of my way,' Bob says, eyes flashing, determined to teach Phil a lesson.

'I can't let you do that,' I say, standing my ground.

Bob looks me up and down wildly. For a moment I think he's going to strike, but he doesn't. Then he starts muttering something about fascist thugs and settles himself back down shakily in his chair.

'If you want to help him, get him a new brain,' Phil says from behind me.

The salty smell of gravy wafts into the bay. 'I think lunch is coming,' I say.

Eventually Bob is moved to another bay to reduce the risk of friction with Phil. One day I go to tell him that his niece is applying to get funding for a nursing home place via a charitable grant and I find him sitting in his chair under a faded print of bright yellow sunflowers. He is sobbing silently, tears running down his face. Outside snow is gently cloaking the grey town.

'Where am I?' he says, clutching my arm. 'What the hell is this place?'

I explain calmly where he is.

'I don't understand,' he says, tears tumbling down his cheeks, down his upper lip and into his mouth. 'Why am I here?'

Once again I explain that we're waiting until his home situation is sorted out.

He looks at me pleadingly. 'Please can you get me out of here?'

'Soon,' I say, patting his hand. I can feel that he's trembling.

'Where's Daisy?' he asks.

'Who's Daisy?'

Now the tears are pouring and through choking sobs Bob says, 'My fiancée.'

'I don't know where she is,' I say. 'I'll go and look for her in a minute if you'd like.'

This seems to calm him. 'Please,' he says.

'Where did you meet?' I ask, trying to soothe him through his memories.

'Doug introduced us at the YMCA charity ball; she was the first person I ever danced with.' He is smiling through the tears. 'She taught me how to jitterbug . . .' He tails off.

'Right,' I say, watching the snow slowly obscure the pathways and roads around the hospital, the sodium lamps glowing into life; it's still only late afternoon.

'What does Daisy look like?' I ask.

His mouth opens as if to answer and then he stops himself. His cheeks droop and he begins sobbing again. 'I don't remember,' he says.

I pat his hand. 'Don't worry, I'll find her for you,' I repeat to him and stand up.

He looks up at me suspiciously. Something has clicked and he is no longer convinced by my play-acting. Quite rightly he doesn't trust me.

'I need to get out of here,' Bob says through the tears, agitated now. He pushes my arm away and begins to stand up.

'Not now, Bob,' I say.

'I need to get out,' he screams at me, trying to push me aside.

'Bob, you're in hospital, remember; you need to stay.'

Jacob, a large black nurse, comes to stand behind me.

'Come on, Bob, have a sit-down and I'll get you a cup of tea,' he says.

'Fuck off, you black bastard,' Bob says.

'You mustn't speak to Jacob like that,' I say firmly.

Jacob laughs. 'Don't worry about it,' he says. 'Bob doesn't mean it. We're friends.'

Something in Jacob's tone settles Bob and with a sob he staggers backwards and slumps in his chair. Jacob draws him a cup of tea from the trolley and I leave them to it.

When I look back a few minutes later Bob is lying asleep, snoring gently, with his head resting on Jacob's massive shoulder. Night has fallen. The size difference makes Bob look like a young boy snoozing against his father. Or Jacob like a boy with a rag doll.

Another morning when we come in, Bob is still lying in his bed, half asleep, muttering to himself, sweat across his brow.

'We've just done the obs and he's got a fever,' Jacob tells me.

I examine him and from the crackles on his chest it's clear that he's picked up a chest infection. For a few days he is quite sick and needs intravenous fluids and antibiotics. The ward is a much quieter place with him ill in bed and all of us ward staff are sombre at the thought of him dying.

'He'll pull through,' Jacob says to me confidentially, then he turns to Bob. 'You're a tough guy, ain't you, Bob?' But I can see the worry in Jacob's face.

I call in Bob's niece and explain how sick he is and the limits of care that we have set for him. The prospect of his death makes her reflective. She's very fond of Bob, though they weren't particularly close, she says; he wouldn't let people get close as he was always quite private and self-contained. Starting when she was a kid and until last year Bob would come over for Christmas dinner with her and her family every year without fail, but he never wanted to stay the night. He and his brother – her father, Derek – were adopted out by a mother they never knew and into an unaffectionate family, as far as she could tell from the little her father said. She thinks that's why they were such private men. They worked together in a bakery business. Bob looked up to Derek, and Derek thrived on Bob's respect. When Bob went away to Manchester for a year to try to expand the business Derek seemed slightly broken, she says. When he came back they both seemed relieved.

'Did you ever hear of a Daisy?' I ask.

'No,' she says. 'Why? Who is she?'

'Bob talked about her,' I say. 'An old flame, I think.'

'Never heard of her,' she says thoughtfully. 'He never had a girlfriend or partner that I knew of, never spoke about things. He was private like I said.'

'He's the last of that generation in my family,' she says. 'It's going to be strange not to have any of them around.'

Bob begins to improve. The fevers go away. He begins eating and drinking, sitting out in his chair. One morning he upbraids me for the creases in my shirt.

'They'll laugh at you if you don't scrub up,' he says, still weak from his pneumonia. 'You don't wanna give 'em the chance.'

'I'll try to do better,' I say, wondering who 'they' are. 'It's good to have you back, Bob.'

For some reason I hold out my hand and we shake.

'Daft bugger,' he says.

*

The next morning I come in to find a plump sweaty woman with a mop of dyed-red hair lying in Bob's bed under the bright yellow sunflowers. It triggers a memory of the day Bob replaced Janet and I feel my pulse speeding up and my stomach churning when I think what had happened to her. I turn to Sally who's sitting at the nurse's station finishing her notes from the night shift and point at the bed. 'Bob?'

She sees my face and smiles. 'A step-down bed in the Lilacs Nursing Home came free yesterday evening and they took him straight over.'

I take a deep breath. 'Thank God for that.'

Sally reads my mind. 'He was fit and happy and raring to go.'

'I'll bet,' I say. 'Is it a good place, the Lilacs?'

'Yes,' Sally says. 'It's not bad. Better equipped for someone like Bob.'

I think back over Bob's time here: all the distress, all the arguments, all the moving, almost killing him with the chest infection, just because no one can work out who should pay for a bed that costs a fraction of this one. He may be demented but who is more crazy? What sort of society promises to help the most vulnerable but never gets around to it, while the suffering goes on and on?

'I'll miss him,' I say. 'For four months he's been the life and soul of this place.'

Sally laughs. 'Don't worry. He said he'd be back to check on us, said he'd been in business too long to leave the lunatics running the asylum.'

Bunker

The elderly man walks gingerly across the room and lowers himself carefully on to the chair and once safely there beams at me.

We start off by talking about the inclement weather and the number of homeless people on the street. Clive tells me that he misses his wife, but that he sees a lot of his son who lives nearby. Every day he walks to his local pub, has a pint, some food, chats with the bartender and other regulars about politics, local news, the football.

When I ask him how he's feeling, he says fine.

'Just the same as ever,' he says. 'Perhaps the knee's more creaky.'

'And you've decided against treatment?' I ask, referring to the cancer that we discovered in his prostate, lymph nodes and bones.

'Yeah, well, something's got to take me,' he says with a smile. 'It's in there but what can I do about it? There's plenty in there that I can't do nothing about.'

I ask whether he understands the options. He gives me the details and it's the usual conundrum: a combination of surgery, chemo and radiotherapy could buy him time, but the time would be unpleasant.

'I'm not afraid of death,' he says simply. 'Pain's another matter, but the cancer doc said they could give me stuff for that if it came to it.'

'I'm sorry it took us so long to get the diagnosis,' I say. 'I'm not really sure what happened there. I can see that we found the first symptoms in January, did the prostate examination and got the blood test that showed there might be something up, but then there's a long gap until we got you diagnosed.'

He chuckles. 'No need to apologize. Not at all. It was my fault really.'

'What do you mean?'

'I got a letter saying they wanted me to have an MRI scan.'

'Yes,' I say.

'And I didn't answer their letter. Then you guys were on at me too and I didn't get back to you either.'

'Oh.' We sit there in silence. 'Sometimes people prefer not to know what's going on inside them,' I say.

His eyes glint and he smiles. 'Afraid, you mean?'

'Well . . .'

'I wasn't worried about what they would find,' he says, 'not that.'

And then, for some reason, he starts describing a scene from his childhood, when he was about eight years old, and walking carefree around the country lanes with his mates during the holidays. He was always the bravest one, wanting to roam the furthest from home, climbing to the highest, thinnest branches in the trees, the first to jump off bridges into the river. And one day they came across a small square entrance in a half-buried concrete structure and assumed it was some sort of Second World War bunker and this old man, as a boy, decided he wanted to see what was inside, and as he's describing this wish I can see a ghost of that ancient enthusiasm settle on his face.

'So I tried to crawl in,' he tells me all those years later.

'Well, I kind of went arms first, and it was dark and smelly and quite steep downwards, and then I got halfway in and all of a sudden I realized I couldn't move, either forward or back.'

He chuckles now at the plight of his youthful self. 'The concrete was tight round my shoulders, and I couldn't see a thing, my own body blocking out the light, and I wriggled with all my might and tried to get a foothold with my toes but could not move an inch.'

He's animated telling the tale, boyish, the gulf of eighty years bridged with one flight of memory.

'And, you know what, I can still remember the smell of that place now. It stank of earth, it was sour and there was another smell in there too, something hard to place, but I got it into my young head that it was the smell of death.'

At this the old man pauses as some emotion rushes in and he has to swallow before he carries on. 'And I suddenly got the feeling that I was never going to get out of there and I began to panic. I wanted to shout out but then I got frightened about what might be further down inside hearing me. The thought of some sort of creature, coming out towards me was . . .'

The man, quieter now, in awe of the feeling, cannot finish the sentence. His eyes are bulging a little in his face.

'So I just began frantically kicking my legs, going mad with fear, keeping completely silent, trying not to wake the beast or whatever it was.'

He laughs now at the memory, safe all these years later in a well-lit room.

'It seemed like I was stuck down there for ages and the outside world had disappeared. And then I felt my mates grabbing me by the ankles, and after a bit they managed to pull me out.'

His old lined face relaxes and he smiles again. 'I tell you, I can still remember now just lying there after they got me out into the sunlight, the sense of relief as I felt the warm breeze on my face, the fresh smell of the wood, the sound of the birds, the sight of the spring leaves on the trees dancing above me.'

He turns and looks at me meaningfully. 'I could never handle a tight space after that. That's why the scanner was impossible for me. That's why it took so long to find out about the cancer.'

'Oh,' I say. 'I see.'

'When someone finally got hold of me and they explained they could diagnose it a different way I went for that.'

I look at Clive – the clumps of cancer slowly gnawing away at his innards – and wonder how much of a difference the delay made. No one will ever know.

'I've had a good innings,' he says, as if in answer to my thoughts. 'Yes, I have.'

I look for the eight-year-old boy in the man sitting there in the chair with his stiff fragile legs, the thin strands of hair combed across his head, the large ears and pendulous nose, tremulous hands, skin dotted with spots, lumps and veins.

And then he's off, back into his life. And I see the boyish excitement and pride back on his face. Telling me stories about work, about falling in love, the children, the disap-pointments, the victories, all the bits that are important to him. The accidents that directed him on his long journey.

Murmur

'We are all dying,' our consultant Dr Esfahani likes to remind us, 'but some are dying more quickly than others.' At the top of a grey 1970s tower block on the edge of a grey town in the middle of England perches the geriatrics ward. This ward is where the more rapidly dying people of this town come.

This morning the medical ward round – eight of us in total from consultant to medical student – stands outside a side room chaotic with fatigue, stress, hangover, hunger, future plans and ambitions. Side rooms are kept for the infectious, dying or for private payers. Dr Esfahani tells the rest of the round to continue to the next patient and takes me into the room with him.

To one side of the hospital the town bustles with the morning commute: a fretwork of roads and cycle lanes cor-ralling the commuters, schoolchildren and ambulances on to the business of their day. The window of the small side room looks the other way over vast fields of wheat and barley awaiting harvest, and, in the distance, gigantic pylons and the motorway snaking away across the country.

Light from the high window floods on to the occupant of the bed: a woman, 103 years old. She is tiny, birdlike, dwarfed by the anonymous sky-blue hospital gown. Her eyes are closed. She is breathing heavily. She is sleeping or dying, I still cannot tell which, but her face is unlined by pain or anx-iety. When the door to the room shuts out the hubbub of the ward outside, Dr Esfahani puts his finger to his lips and says, 'Listen.'

I do and I can hear a swooshing sound coming from the tiny chest of the lady in the bed before us. The swooshing noise is in time with every heartbeat. Behind her ribcage, which is prominent through her hospital gown, sits the heart muscle that has tapped out the duration of her stay on this planet from her brief holiday inside her mother's womb in 1911 until these last days. Quickening with activity, fear, lust; slowing for the duration of her 100,000 meals, her 35,000 sleeps. Now there is a regurgitation of blood through a leaky heart valve. With every wave the tide drags back on the pebbles.

The loose mitral valve means that her heart is now struggling to get sufficient blood to the peripheries of her body for them to function properly, including her brain. Any small increase in exertion, passion or even a common cold, could make the blood requirements outstrip the amounts. This is probably the cause of her collapse, the thing that, we can see from the notes, frightened her carers and made them call an ambulance. The thing that has brought her from her care home surrounded by the elderly, gardens and peace to this small top-of-the-tower, light-washed room, this hive of medicine. At any moment her heart could give out. Her precarious balance on the cusp of life is audible from the end of the bed.

Dr Esfahani smiles ruefully. 'Why is she here?' he whispers.

I leaf through the folder of notes I am clutching and quietly read out the results of the blood tests, heart tracing and head scan she had in A & E last night, all of which are in keeping with being 103 years old.

The consultant gently cuts me off. 'Why is she here?' he repeats quietly.

We are still away from the bed by the door. We are talking so there is no way the patient can hear us.

'Is she a candidate for valve surgery?' he asks.

We look at the long list of her co-morbidities on her notes then across to the patient. She is very frail. The correct answer is clearly no.

'What if it gave her one extra day?' I ask, playing devil's advocate.

Dr Esfahani smiles. 'It would be more likely to take away her last day.'

The light in the room is greyer now as a large cumulonimbus cloud drifts across the sky.

'Any family?' he asks.

I've already checked. The next of kin boxes are all blank. The only clues we have to her life are her name, her date of birth and a list of medical problems.

'Hello, Mrs Abbott,' Dr Esfahani says loudly, approaching the bed. She smiles at the sound but does not open her eyes.

He gently examines her with hands and stethoscope. While he does so I wonder at Mrs Abbot's life. From the horse and cart to the space and computer age. Two world wars, loss of empire, the disappearance of God, flower power, the shrinkage of the globe. What did she do during this long existence? Did she have parents, brothers, sisters, friends, lovers, children? Did she work? In an office, on a farm, as a seamstress, an engineer? Does anyone alive know? Is that life carried somewhere in her? Does any of it matter?

Dr Esfahani ushers me to listen through the stethoscope.

The murmur is deafening in my ears and her heart kicks the bones of her ribcage into my hand with each beat.

We step away from the bed to the window. He dictates his simple findings to me.

'Where does she live?'

I name the care home and he nods. 'It's a nice place,' he says.

'What shall we do, Tom?'

'Get her home,' I say.

He nods again then turns and looks out of the window over the fields.

'Have you heard of the poet Hafiz?' he asks me. I am surprised as he has scarcely mentioned anything unrelated to medicine in the three months we have worked together.

'Yes,' I say.

'I used to know some of his poems by heart,' he says. 'I would visit my grandmother in Tehran when I was a kid. She made me learn them.'

The large cloud has drifted on and sunlight floods us through the glass once again. We look out over the heart of England. In the distance the pylons and the motorway stretch twinkling and gleaming as far as the eye can see. A strong wind ruffles the barley below.

'*I saw the green meadow of the sky and the sickle moon, and remembered my own life's field and the time of harvest,*' he says gently.

A plane slits the sky, carrying passengers to lands unknown.

Dr Esfahani turns back and we look at the woman lying in the bed. 'Mrs Abbot,' he says, 'we are going to get you home.'

Epilogue

That last patient takes me back many years to my first job as a newly qualified doctor in geriatrics. Winter was approaching and things were frenetic. I know that Mrs Abbot left the ward later that day. As to what exactly happened to her next, and to most of the patients in this book, I have no idea. But her GP would have known. They are at the heart of things, the hub of the patient's medical life, the first and last port of call. They get to write and read more chapters of a patient's story than anyone else in medicine.

And that was the speciality I decided to pursue. Now on a daily basis I see pregnant women, young babies, children with fevers, tormented teenagers, students with sports and drinking injuries, workers and parents balancing chronic illnesses with the demands of their lives, the middle-aged with their heart attacks and cancer diagnoses, old-age joint problems and dementia, and those late home visits to prescribe palliative medicines.

Last year we added a new disease to the long list. With the advent of the Covid-19 pandemic our common human frailty has been rammed home. Like the virus, we have had to adapt. We start each consultation on the phone, the patient a disembodied voice, whose tone is as useful a guide as the words that are spoken. We carefully choose who needs to be seen and touched in person. Now we do most of our work in masks, aprons and gloves – new barriers between the doctor and patient to which again we must adapt.

It is still a rich and fulfilling job. Thousands of patients a year flow through the surgery and together we wind our complex journeys from birth to death.

Endnotes on the Diseases

Snow in May

One in every 250 pregnancies ends in a **stillbirth** (loss of life after twenty-four weeks' gestation but before birth) and every day eight women in the UK give birth to a stillborn baby.

Forty per cent of stillbirths happen due to infection, problems with the placenta, congenital abnormality, foetal growth restriction or complications with twins. The other 60% are unexplained.

Women who suffer a stillbirth have higher than average rates of depression, anxiety and PTSD.

As well as stillbirth, one in four women will experience a miscarriage (loss of pregnancy in the first twenty-three weeks of gestation) and 1 in every 350 pregnancies ends in neonatal death (death in the first twenty-eight days of life).

Research continues to try to understand the causes, and to develop practices to reduce the risks of miscarriage, stillbirth and neonatal death.

Support group:
Tommy's (www.tommys.org)

Rap Birth

Newborn babies are exceptionally vulnerable to abuse and neglect, and pregnancy can be an extremely stressful and emotionally complex time for parents. The decision to place newborns in care is incredibly difficult for parents and professionals. Roughly 1 in 300 newborns (aged 0–7 days) in England are taken into care, an average of seven every day of the year. It is not clear what proportion of these 'care proceedings' are initiated by the parents. Only 10% of these children will end up back living with their mothers.

Vulnerable parents should get support during pregnancy, but if concerns about the newborn's safety are sufficiently high by the time of birth a court order may be sought to have the baby removed from the parent. Substance misuse and mental health issues can be the triggers for such safeguarding proceedings. These removals have an acutely distressing effect on mothers, fathers and the broader family, as well as the professionals involved.

Support group:
Family Lives (www.familylives.org.uk)

Hunger

Every year around eight million infants (6% of worldwide births) are born with a serious birth defect of genetic or partially genetic origin. Although rare at 1 in every 15,000 live births, **Prader–Willi syndrome** is one of the better understood genetic syndromes. It occurs because of a loss of function of the genes on the fifteenth chromosome. It is usually inherited through a complex (and fascinating) genetic process known as genomic imprinting.

Every person with Prader–Willi syndrome is unique, but the core characteristics of the condition are that as newborns they have weak muscle tone, feeding difficulties, poor growth and delayed development. Then in childhood they develop an insatiable appetite, which leads to chronic overeating. If unchecked, this can cause obesity and related health problems. Other common features of Prader–Willi syndrome are mild to moderate intellectual impairment and learning disabilities, distinctive facial characteristics, low self-esteem and depression.

Parents of children with Prader–Willi syndrome often have to manage challenging behaviour. But the core task for parents and caregivers remains restricting children to a low-calorie diet and encouraging regular exercise. Fridges and cupboards at home often end up padlocked. All of this, and uncertainty about their child's future, can result in significant carer fatigue.

Support group:
Prader–Willi Syndrome Association UK (www.pwsa.co.uk/services)

Oxygen

Anaphylaxis is a severe and potentially life-threatening allergic reaction. Recent data suggests that the incidence is increasing and 0.5–2% of us will suffer from it at least once in our lifetimes. Deaths from anaphylaxis are exceedingly rare but, because it can be hard to distinguish severe from mild reactions, it should always be treated promptly.

Allergic reactions occur when the immune system 'over-reacts' to a substance inhaled, ingested or placed on the skin, and releases chemicals that cause symptoms such as a rash or itching in the nose. In anaphylactic reactions the same process happens but in more than one part of the body at the same time. It typically occurs rapidly (minutes to hours) after the patient has been exposed to a food, medicine, insect bite or other trigger, and requires rapid treatment with adrenaline to mitigate the most deadly effects. Antihistamines and steroids are also commonly given.

Anaphylaxis classically causes a nettle-like rash or swelling of the face or mouth, as well as tightening of the airways, low blood pressure and a fast heart rate. The patient might feel faint, nauseous, breathless and/or anxious. In a minority of cases – like ours with Solveig – many of these symptoms are absent and it can become harder to diagnose and distinguish from other illnesses.

Support group:
Allergy UK (www.allergyuk.org)

Diplomat

Defining what counts as a **mental health disorder** is extremely difficult. According to the World Health Organization, mental disorders 'are generally characterized by some combination of abnormal thoughts, emotions, behaviour and relationships with others'. To be classified as a disorder these 'abnormalities' have to cause either significant distress or impairment in functioning.

A recent rigorous survey on the mental health of children and young people in England, found that one in eight (13%) five- to nineteen-year-olds were suffering from at least one mental health disorder, and that one in twenty (5%) suffered from at least two mental health disorders. (Other studies suggest these and the following figures may be an underestimate.) Of those in the survey the majority (around 8% of all children) were suffering from an 'emotional disorder' (anxiety, depression or bipolar disorder). Around 5% suffered from behavioural disorders (characterized by repetitive and persistent patterns of disruptive and violent behaviour in which the rights of others, and social norms or rules, are violated), 2% suffered from hyperactivity disorders, another 1% suffered from an autism spectrum disorder, and another 1% suffered from one of a series of less common disorders (tics, eating disorders, mutism, psychosis). Only one in four of these children had contact with a mental health specialist.

The same survey found that one out of every twenty preschool children suffered from a mental health disorder: mainly behavioural, autistic spectrum or related to sleeping or feeding.

Categories of children who were more likely to suffer from a mental health disorder included those who have a physical health problem or special educational needs, being white British, not identifying as heterosexual, coming from a low-income household, having a family member with their own mental health problems and using social media on a daily basis.

As transgender issues have gained increased recognition in recent years they have become a source of growing controversy. According to the World Health Organization, 'Transgender is an umbrella term that describes a diverse group of people whose internal sense of gender is different than that which they were assigned at birth. Transgender refers to gender identity and gender expression, and has nothing to do with sexual orientation.'

Support groups:
Mental Health Foundation (www.mentalhealth.org.uk); Young Minds (www.youngminds.org.uk); Gender Identity Clinic (www.gic.nhs.uk/info-support)

Happiness

About one in a thousand babies are born with **Down's syndrome** each year in the UK. People with Down's syndrome are born with a full or partial extra copy of chromosome 21 (people usually have two of each chromosome); this alters the course of their physical development and causes characteristics associated with Down's.

Common physical traits include a single deep crease across the palm, an upward slant to the eyes, a smaller than usual mouth and stature, and low muscle tone. Most children with Down's have some level of learning disability. People with Down's are more likely than average to suffer from certain heart, stomach, sight and hearing problems, and from certain cancers.

There are around 40,000 people in the UK living with Down's syndrome. Though many of them are able to work and choose to do so, there is significant underemployment among people with Down's (as with other learning disabilities).

Cancer is the joint-biggest killer of five- to fourteen-year-olds globally, roughly equalling the numbers who die from road accidents. In Britain almost 2,000 children are diagnosed with cancer every year. The types of cancers that develop in children are often different from those that develop in adults. Cancers of the bone marrow and blood (leukaemia) and of the brain and spinal cord are the most common childhood cancers (accounting for over half of the total). Children with Down's syndrome have a significantly higher risk of developing leukaemia in childhood in comparison to other children.

Around three quarters of children diagnosed with cancer in the UK survive their disease for ten years or more, though the odds vary with different types of cancer.

A cancer diagnosis and its treatment can have significant long-term physical effects for the patient that last into adulthood, along with vast psychological effects for patients, their families and their friends.

Support groups:
Down's Syndrome Association (www.downs-syndrome.org.uk); and for getting into work, Workfit (www.dsworkfit.org.uk)

Cancer Research (https://www.cancerresearchuk.org/about-cancer/childrens-cancer/support-organisations/organisations)

Aztec Priest

Suicide is the single biggest killer of men under forty-five in the UK, the single biggest killer of twenty- to thirty-four-year-olds of both sexes in this country and the second leading cause of death among fifteen- to twenty-nine-year-olds globally. Suicide accounted for 794,000 deaths globally in 2017, more than those dying from all other forms of violence (war, murder, terrorism, execution) put together.

The annual suicide rate per 100,000 people ranges from two in Kuwait to fifty in Greenland. The UK incidence in 2018 was 11 per 100,000, accounting for 6,507 deaths.

The suicide rate has been declining globally over the last twenty years and in the UK there has been a gradual decline in suicides since the late 1980s, but in 2018 the numbers increased by 12%. There was a change in the way this data was collected part way through the year but this does not seem to explain the full extent of the increase. Rates among under-twenty-fives have generally increased in recent years. Three quarters of UK suicides are among men. Suicidal acts are extremely complex, and numerous cultural, social, psychological and physical factors can contribute to them. Factors that reduce vulnerability to suicide include being in full-time employment or a supportive school environment and having strong social connections.

Suicide-bereaved families suffer from higher levels of rejection, shame, stigma and blame than those bereaved in other ways. Family and friends of people who have taken their own life suffer higher rates of depression, PTSD and suicidal thinking. Counselling, family therapy, complicated grief therapy and support groups have all been shown to help those bereaved by suicide.

Support if suicidal:
NHS 111 (phone 111); your GP; Samaritans (phone 116 123, email jo@samaritans.org); CALM (Campaign Against Living Miserably) from 5 p.m. to midnight, helpline (0800 585858) or webchat (www.thecalmzone.net/help/webchat); Papyrus (for young people up to the age of thirty-five who are worried about how they are feeling or anyone concerned about a young person) phone 0800 068 4141, text 07860 039967 or email pat@papyrus-uk.org.

Resources to support after a suicide:
Survivors of Bereavement by Suicide (0300 111 5065; www.uksobs.org); Support After Suicide Partnership (www.supportaftersuicide.org.uk); www.nhs.uk/Livewell/Suicide/Documents/Help is at Hand.pdf

Female. 18. Back Pain.

Denied pregnancy – when a woman is unaware of or unable to accept the fact she is pregnant – and concealed pregnancy – when a woman hides her pregnancy – are rare. It is often hard to distinguish between the two. One German study found that 1 in 500 pregnancies were denied at twenty weeks gestation, and 1 in 2,500 pregnancies were denied throughout pregnancy until the point of labour starting. This suggests that many of those who initially deny pregnancy eventually acknowledge it and come to terms with it.

It used to be thought that women who denied pregnancy tended to be young, in first pregnancy, often with learning difficulties, mental health conditions or a history of substance abuse. But a more recent study looking at the characteristics of sixty-five randomly selected women who denied pregnancy found them to have a wide range of backgrounds and characteristics. The median age was twenty-seven years, 63% had a partner and forty-four had been pregnant before. Only three had schizophrenia and only one was a substance misuser.

Another study found that: 'The absence of many physical symptoms of pregnancy, inexperience, general inattentiveness to bodily cues, intense psychological conflicts about the pregnancy, and external stresses can contribute to the denial in otherwise well-adjusted women.'

Outcomes for the mothers and babies of denied pregnancies are statistically more likely than the average pregnancy to end with emotional disturbance of the mother, abuse, neglect or neonaticide. But many women are said to 'reconstitute' their denial on giving birth and take full responsibility for their infants.

Support group:
Best Beginnings (https://www.bestbeginnings.org.uk)

The Outsider

The thyroid is a butterfly-shaped gland located in the neck. It produces hormones that regulate many processes within our bodies. Too little thyroid hormone and many functions of the cells and organs of the body slow down; too much, as with Tariq, and they speed up.

Thyrotoxicosis affects around 2% of UK women and 0.2% of UK men. It results from excess levels of circulating thyroid hormones, which can cause fluctuations in weight, appetite and periods in women, diarrhoea, sweating, tremor, heat intolerance, heart palpitations and mental illness.

The majority of such cases (80%) are caused by the immune system attacking the thyroid gland. Rarely they are caused by problems, including tumours, of the pituitary gland, which is responsible for stimulating the work of the thyroid gland.

Support group:
British Thyroid Foundation (www.btf-thyroid.org)

Transmission

Since it emerged in the late 1970s **HIV/AIDS** has killed an estimated 32 million people worldwide.

The human immunodeficiency virus targets several types of cell in the immune system and as the virus proliferates, over a matter of years, the body loses the capability to defend itself against certain infections. Transmission can occur through sexual contact, through blood sharing (usually via needles in drug users), and from pregnant mothers to their unborn children.

When the HIV/AIDS pandemic struck in the early 1980s patients began developing strange illnesses that doctors rarely saw, like the fungal chest infection PCP that Nick had.

Only people with immune systems that were heavily suppressed by chemotherapy or damaged in the specific manner of a longstanding HIV infection can develop these particular infections and cancers, and they became known as 'AIDS-defining illnesses'.

Prior to 1994 a third of those diagnosed with HIV in the UK died from the disease. Since then the development of highly active antiretroviral treatment and earlier diagnosis of the disease, so that cases are caught before the immune system is severely suppressed, mean patient outcomes have massively improved. Now people diagnosed early with HIV and on effective treatment have a comparable life expectancy to people the same age who do not have the disease. It is now rare in the UK to see someone in Nick's position.

In the UK in 2018 an estimated 103,800 people were living with HIV. 93% of these knew they had HIV, 97% of those who knew were on treatment, and of these 97% were virally suppressed (which meant they could not pass the virus on).

If high-risk individuals without HIV take pre-exposure prophylaxis (PrEP) antiretroviral medication four times a week, their risk of contracting the disease, even when having sex with infected individuals, is reduced by 99%. PrEP is widely available on the NHS in Scotland and Wales, and should now be available in England through sexual health clinics, and in Northern Ireland you can enrol on a study to access the drug (www.iwantprepnow.co.uk).

Support groups:
National AIDS Trust (www.nat.org.uk); Positively UK (www.positivelyuk.org)

The Bent Knife

There are 2.5 million **violent incidents** in England and Wales annually, resulting in 300,000 A & E attendances and 35,000 emergency hospital admissions. The most deprived communities have five times the rate of violence-related hospital admissions than the most affluent.

People aged sixteen to twenty-four run the highest risk of being victims of violent crime, with an equal split between offences carried out by strangers and offences by acquaintances.

Knives are the most common instrument used in murders, but only account for 6% of violent assaults. There were 20,000 **stabbings** in England and Wales, leading to over 5,000 hospital admissions, 235 murders and 412 attempted murders in the latest recorded year. One in four of those murdered were men aged eighteen to twenty-four.

The risk factors for people to become perpetrators of violence are many and complex. They include neglect and abuse in childhood, poor family functioning, domestic violence in the home, delinquent peers, living in a high-crime area, personality traits and social inequality. Almost half of all violence is committed by people under the influence of alcohol. Research shows violence can be contagious. Children exposed to violence early in life are more likely to be violent as adults. They are also more likely to suffer from substance abuse, obesity, cancer and heart disease in later life. Violence inhibits community cohesion and impacts on community mental well-being and quality of life, preventing people from using outdoor space and public transport.

The most successful interventions target parents and children in at-risk families and promote positive behaviours that can transform lives. These include the Family Nurse Partnership programme and the Sure Start Children's Centres, social development and anti-bullying programmes in schools, community-based programmes and intervention work with at-risk adolescents and those already in gangs.

Support group:
Victim Support (www.victimsupport.org.uk)

The Lady in the Bed

It was not possible to diagnose Kevin from our brief encounter but he seems to have been suffering from some sort of **somatic symptom disorder**. These are a group of illnesses for all of which the patient experiences symptoms that are not borne out by medical investigation or logic. In somatic symptom disorder there is an underlying illness but the symptoms experienced by the patient seem far more severe than the underlying problem warrants. In conversion disorder the patient experiences symptoms of the nerves affecting movement or the senses (i.e. weakness, seizures, numbness) with no apparent underlying damage. In factitious disorder symptoms are fabricated or the patients secretly harm themselves. In all these illnesses the patient gains some sort of psychological reward from seeing medical professionals but is not seeking monetary gain.

Subarachnoid haemorrhages are rare types of strokes that are notable for their high mortality rate and for affecting younger patients. They tend to occur in people who have small swellings in one of the arteries in the brain. These swellings can burst, and when they do they bleed into the brain at high pressure, causing a sudden-onset headache and, often, other symptoms. In around half of cases the pressure damages the parts of the brain that keep the heart pumping and the lungs breathing, killing the patient.

Support groups:
Mind (www.mind.org.uk)
Stroke Association (www.stroke.org.uk)

Joker

Traumatic brain injury (TBI) is the commonest cause of death and disability in people aged one to forty in the UK, and every year 1.4 million patients in England and Wales attend hospital following a head injury.

Falls and road traffic accidents are the most frequent causes. Assaults account for around 30% of all TBI in those aged twenty to thirty. Penetrating brain injuries, as in Sonny's case, are rare, especially off the battlefield.

Improvements in managing TBI in hospital and better motor vehicle safety design have resulted in better survival rates. Unfortunately the majority of survivors of moderate and severe TBI are left with brain damage that leads to long-term physical, psychological and behavioural problems. These affect the patient's ability to readapt to independent living, work, social and family life, and can have profoundly distressing effects on their family and friends.

The outcomes of the damage depend on which parts of the brain suffered the damage. Cognitive problems include poor attention, memory, impulse control, information processing and speech and language. Personality changes can include high levels of impulsivity and anger, and wild and deep swings in mood. Patients often are not aware, or only slightly aware, of these changes. Patients with TBI are more at risk of suffering from depression, anxiety or psychosis.

Rehabilitation can be painstaking, arduous but can sometimes lead to significant improvement. **Witzelsucht** or 'wise-cracking syndrome' can be seen in some sufferers of TBI and also in certain forms of dementia.

Support group:
Headway (www.headway.org.uk)

Smile

Multiple sclerosis is a chronic, progressive illness that affects the brain and spinal cord. Over 100,000 people in the UK have multiple sclerosis and it affects three times as many women as men.

The patient's immune system attacks the layer that protects and insulates nerve fibres; this disrupts the ability of the nervous system to send signals around the body, leading to a wide range of symptoms.

Different patients get different symptoms at different times. Multiple sclerosis can affect balance; speech and swallowing; limb stiffness and tremor; vision; fatigue; pins and needles; cramps and pain; bladder and bowel function; memory, thinking and emotional control.

Some people get the disease mildly; others much more

severely. Most people are diagnosed between the ages of twenty and fifty. The disease tends to progress, causing more problems over time, but the rate of this deterioration can be very variable. If untreated, more than 30% of patients will have significant disability within twenty to twenty-five years of disease onset. There are medications that can help reduce the rate of progression for some patients and there are lifestyle adaptations (such as electric wheelchairs, home modifications, gastrostomy tubes) and therapies that can help the patient live as full a life as possible.

Living with a progressive incurable disease can take a huge psychological toll on sufferers and their families and friends. In the end stages the symptoms become more severe and disabling.

Support group:
Multiple Sclerosis Society (www.mssociety.org.uk)

Gash

In the UK 27% of those who kill themselves have seen their GP in the previous week. Most people who die by suicide have not attempted it before. Most people who have **attempted suicide** will never make a successful attempt. One review of long-term studies found that 70% made no further attempts, 23% reattempted non-fatally and 7% eventually died by suicide. Another study found that 1–2% of those who attempted suicide would succeed in killing themselves within a year.

Identifying those who will reattempt is exceedingly difficult.

The first six months after the initial attempts are believed to be the most risky. Previous attempts with high intent to kill are more predictive of future attempts. Being male, unemployed, living alone, unmarried, dependent on drugs or alcohol and having active mental illness or having ease of access to means of suicide are all thought to increase the risk. The evidence is weak, but protective factors may include religious faith, having children at home, family support, problem-solving skills and a sense of responsibility to others.

One study found that 'recent disruption of a relationship with a partner and major rows rarely preceded the attempts of those who later killed themselves'.

Support if suicidal:
NHS 111 (phone 111); your GP; Samaritans (phone 116 123, email jo@samaritans.org); CALM (Campaign Against Living Miserably) from 5 p.m. to midnight, helpline (0800 585858) or webchat (www.thecalmzone. net/help/webchat); Papyrus (for young people up to the age of thirty-five who are worried about how they are feeling or anyone concerned about a young person) phone 0800 068 4141, text 07860 039967 or email pat@ papyrus-uk.org.

Resources to support after a suicide:
Survivors of Bereavement by Suicide (0300 111 5065; www.uksobs.org); Support After Suicide Partnership (www.supportaftersuicide.org.uk); www.nhs.uk/Livewell/ Suicide/Documents/Help is at Hand.pdf

Phoenix

Cardiac arrest is the term used to describe when the heart stops pumping blood around the body. This can occur suddenly in a fit and healthy person, it can occur at a particularly severe stage of a treatable disease, and it will also occur at the end of everybody's life. In some cases immediate resuscitation can restart the heart and lead to years or decades of good-quality life for the patient, but in other cases it can be unsuccessful or lead to a brief period of severe ill health followed by death. Of those who have a cardiac arrest in hospital and have successful resuscitation to restart the heart, only 50% survive to go home from hospital. The underlying health of the patient is a good predictor of who will benefit most from resuscitation. Since the 1970s hospitals and GPs have begun to use Do Not Attempt Cardiopulmonary Resuscitation orders to identify patients that should NOT have resuscitation attempted on them. This can involve difficult conversations with patients and their families, but are often welcomed as well.

Speedy resuscitation for those suffering from cardiac arrest in the community can save huge numbers of lives. Bystanders calling 999, then immediately starting chest compressions and accessing the nearest available defibrillator to give an electric shock to the heart, are the key. However, in only a third of cardiac arrests in the UK do bystanders currently attempt resuscitation. Survival rates in the UK are 7%, whereas in Norway it's 25% (where 73% of bystanders attempt CPR). Denmark's rates of bystander CPR doubled within six years of making resuscitation training mandatory in schools, and their survival rates tripled.

Euthanasia is the act of deliberately ending a person's life to relieve suffering, and assisted suicide is the act of helping or encouraging a person to kill themselves. These are both illegal under English law. In some countries euthanasia and/or doctor-assisted suicide are legal and available. The Netherlands, Luxembourg, Belgium and Canada allow both in cases where a patient is enduring unbearable suffering with no prospect of improvement. Palliative care medicine involves the prevention and relief of suffering – be it physical, psychological or spiritual – in people with life-threatening illness. Within this framework withdrawing life-sustaining treatment in a person's best interests is not considered illegal.

Labyrinth

Othello syndrome (aka pathological jealousy) is a type of delusional disorder. Delusional disorders all involve a person suffering from persistent delusions, against the evidence and their cultural context but in the absence of broader psychotic illness. In Othello syndrome the person has the false absolute certainty of the infidelity of a partner, leading to preoccupation with a partner's sexual unfaithfulness based on unfounded evidence.

Delusional disorders are rare, and are believed to affect only two in every thousand people over a lifetime. Factors associated with delusional disorders include marriage, being employed, low-income status and recent immigration. Delusional disorders are hard to treat (medications and psychological therapy are used). However, evidence suggests around 50% of patients make a full recovery and 80–90% show some improvement.

Over a million people in the UK have **bipolar disorder** (previously known as manic depression). The lifetime prevalence of bipolar disorder is around 2%. People with bipolar disorder have recurrent episodes of extreme, often overwhelming moods: periods of highs and lows that last for weeks or months with periods of relatively normal mood in between.

In the high 'manic' or 'hypomanic' episodes the person might feel euphoric, excited, irritable or agitated, overconfident, untouchable or impervious to harm. They can speak rapidly, struggle to sleep, act in an overly friendly, aggressive or sexual manner, misuse recreational substances and act or spend money recklessly. These are then followed by depressive episodes.

Childhood trauma, genetics and stressful life events are all implicated as potential risk factors for bipolar. There are two peaks of onset: between the ages of fifteen and twenty-four and between the ages of forty-five and fifty-four. It takes an average of nine years to get a correct diagnosis, and is usually a lifelong condition. Although treatment with psychological talking therapies and mood-stabilizing drugs can be very effective, 60% of people with bipolar receive no medical attention at all.

Support group:
Mind (www.mind.org.uk)
Bipolar UK (www.bipolaruk.org)

Octopus Trap

Roughly 150,000 people in the UK suffer from **Parkinson's disease**. Symptoms usually develop in people over the age of fifty. In rare cases symptoms start in people of under forty. Researchers believe that in most individuals the cause is a combination of genetics and environmental exposure.

Parkinson's patients lose nerve cells in a region of the brain called the substantia nigra, leading to a reduction in the important brain chemical dopamine. Dopamine regulates movement in the body and the classical symptoms of Parkinson's are tremors, slow movement and stiff muscles. Parkinson's can also affect balance, smell, sleep, mood and memory.

Treatments include medication and supportive therapies. The disease is usually progressive, with increasing disability as time passes. Psychological distress for sufferers and their family and friends can be significant. However, the average life expectancy for those with Parkinson's is now approaching that of the general population.

Takotsubo cardiomyopathy (aka broken heart syndrome) involves the weakening of the left ventricle of the heart, resulting in a characteristic 'octopus pot' ballooning, as the result of severe emotional or physical stress. Symptoms are the same as for a heart attack. 90% of reported cases are in females aged fifty-eight to seventy-five, and it may account for up to 5% of women suspected of having a heart attack.

Triggers can include illness, violence, accidents, natural disasters or bereavement. Most people recover normal heart function within one to eight weeks with no long-term heart damage.

Support groups:
Parkinson's UK (www.parkinsons.org.uk)
British Heart Foundation (www.bhf.org.uk)

Prison

The average age of death for **prisoners** in England is fifty-six (compared to eighty-three in the general population). Death rates are even higher among ex-prisoners. Risk of death is highest immediately after release and these cases are often linked to substance misuse. Rates of common physical health problems are roughly double those of the general adult population. Rates of mental health problems are hugely overrepresented, with ten times the general population levels of psychosis and four times the levels of depression, anxiety and personality disorder.

A recent parliamentary report found that the UK government is failing in its duty of care towards prisoners. Prisons are overcrowded, poorly maintained and understaffed. Prisoners are locked in their cells most of the time, with one fifth getting only two hours outside the cell on weekdays. Fifty per cent of prisoners fear violence at some time. Rates of death, suicide, self-harm and violence have been climbing to record highs from already high levels. The number of drug deaths in prison is rising.

Recreational drug use is rife, with 30% of male and 42% of female prisoners reporting a drug habit on arrival and a further 10% reporting that they developed a habit within the prison.

Support group:
Rethink Mental Illness (https://www.rethink.org/advice-and-information/rights-restrictions/police-courts-and-prison/healthcare-in-prison/)

Arrhythmia

Coronary heart disease kills 9.4 million people a year worldwide and is the leading cause of death in every country in the world. In the UK 180 people die from it every day and 2.3 million people are living with it.

Smoking, alcohol, diet, obesity, exercise, air pollution and genetics all play a role in cholesterol deposits in the arteries around the heart, causing pain on exertion ('angina') and heart attacks (when a clot blocks an artery, causing damage to the heart muscle). Death rates from coronary heart disease have fallen by over a half in the last fifty years. This is largely due to reductions in smoking and other public health measures, as well as improvements in treatment, including stenting of coronary arteries. The role of long-term stress in coronary heart disease remains unclear.

'VanillaSky' is one of the many brands of synthetic cathinone: a range of laboratory-produced chemical compounds developed to mimic the effects of cocaine and MDMA ('ecstasy'). The effects of taking unregulated drugs are variable, as the actual compounds within the drug can vary wildly, contaminants can harm or kill, and doses are often extremely hard to anticipate and so accidental overdose is common. Most people who take synthetic cathinones do not end up unwell but in some cases they have been associated with arrhythmias, heart attacks and sudden cardiac death. Substance misuse, homelessness and post-traumatic stress disorder are far higher among **combat veterans** than the general population. One study found that it took an average of eleven years for veterans to seek help for health difficulties after leaving the military.

Support groups:
British Heart Foundation (www.bhf.org.uk)
Combat Stress (www.combatstress.org.uk)

The Nest

The average age of death for **homeless** people is forty-four years. The health of Britain's homeless population is generally dire: 73% suffer a physical health problem; 80% a mental health problem; 77% smoke; 40% have drug problems; and 30% alcohol problems. Homeless people use acute NHS services at four times the rate of the general population, often presenting to services late with problems that would have been far simpler to treat earlier on.

A person with a **personality disorder** has chronic, significant and distressing difficulties in the way they think, feel and behave, and in relating to themselves and to others. Several studies have found the prevalence of personality disorder among street homeless populations to be around 80%. Treatment for personality disorder requires rigorous talking or group therapy, something that is very hard to achieve for homeless people.

Support group:
Crisis (www.crisis.org.uk)

Royal Oak

There were 1.1 million alcohol-related admissions to hospital in 2018, including 340,000 where alcohol was the main reason, and 5,843 alcohol-specific deaths in 2017.

Long-term alcohol misuse can affect the heart, liver, pancreas, brain and nervous system, and is a causal factor in over 200 medical conditions. It is a significant risk factor for many cancers and mental health conditions. Statistically it is rated the sixth biggest cause of disability and death in the UK.

In Great Britain 57% of the adult population reported drinking alcohol in the previous week (29 million people), and of these almost a third 'binged' (men drinking eight units or more, women drinking six units or more). 20% of adults said they never drink alcohol. Men, people aged forty-five to sixty-four and those working in managerial and professional occupations, in addition to the highest earners, were most likely to say they drank alcohol in the past week. The numbers are gradually declining over time and those aged twenty to twenty-four were least likely to report drinking alcohol.

Risk factors for alcohol dependence include parental alcohol problems, chronically high anxiety levels, and high alcohol tolerance.

Support group:
Drinkaware (www.drinkaware.co.uk)

Walking

Psychosis is a condition that affects the way the brain processes information, so that a person loses touch with reality, either through hallucinations (hearing or seeing things others can't), delusions (believing certain things that are neither true, plausible nor believed by peers) or disorganized thinking. Psychosis can be a symptom of severe depression, schizophrenia, bipolar disorder, certain personality disorders, delusional disorder or a response to a particularly stressful experience or severe intoxication.

The most common hallucinations experienced in psychotic episodes are those in which the person hears voices that no one else can hear, often talking about them in a denigratory manner. Seeing, smelling and feeling things that are not there are less common. Delusions are often persecutory.

Treatment varies depending on the underlying illness.

Support group:
Mind (www.mind.org.uk)

The End

One in two of us will get **cancer** in our lifetimes. A thousand people in the UK get a cancer diagnosis every day. Almost 500 people die from cancer daily. There are over two million people living with cancer in the UK.

Cancer happens when abnormal cells in our bodies divide in an uncontrolled way due to genetic mutations. If unchecked, this can lead to clumps of cancerous material (tumours) and can also spread through the bloodstream and seed in other parts of the body (metastasis). These tumours often cause damage to the organs where they're located as well as to the circulation, immune, lymphatic and hormonal systems.

There are over 200 different types of cancer, each a distinct illness with wildly varying survival rates. Early diagnosis is one of the keys to survival. Often the hardest to pick up ('silent') cancers are the most deadly. Treatments for many cancers have transformed the outcomes of this disease for the better.

Thirty-eight per cent of cancer cases are considered preventable. Across the range of the disease the most significant preventable risk factors for cancer are smoking, then obesity, UV radiation, occupation, alcohol and low dietary fibre.

Cancer survival rates are improving but the UK still lags behind much of the developed world, partly because of an average later diagnosis.

Support group:
Cancer Research UK (www.cancerresearchuk.org)

Air Crash

Hip fractures are the most common serious injury in older people in the UK and 65,000 people of all ages presented annually with the problem in 2017. They cost the NHS one billion pounds a year.

The majority of fractures are caused by low-impact falls around the home. Speedy operation, usually with a hip replacement implant, is the norm, and the operation has become increasingly successful with good outcomes. Nonetheless, hip fractures are a common cause of death in the elderly with around 7% of people presenting to hospital with a hip fracture dying within thirty days.

Around one in a thousand people with hip implants suffer a further fracture around the prosthetic hip.

Support group:
Age UK (www.ageuk.org.uk)

Four Sisters

Schizophrenia is an illness with which patients suffer from psychotic symptoms (hallucinations, delusions, disordered thinking, emotional apathy, lack of drive, poverty of speech, social withdrawal and self-neglect) for at least a month.

An estimated 1% of us will suffer from schizophrenia at some point in our lifetimes. Schizophrenia usually starts in late adolescence or early adulthood. Serious acute episodes often result in a brief period of hospitalization and the illness accounts for a third of all mental health and social care spending in the UK.

The mainstay of treatment in the UK and most other countries is with antipsychotic medications. Some countries place more emphasis on psychological therapies; CBT, family therapy and art therapy have been shown to work but are poorly resourced in the UK.

Only a quarter of sufferers will have recovered after five years, but for most people the condition gradually improves over their lifetime, though it is very often associated with poor outcomes in education, work and social parts of life.

An increased risk of suicide and poor physical health means that people with schizophrenia die an average ten to twenty years earlier than the general population.

Support group:
Living With Schizophrenia (www.livingwithschizophre-niauk.org)

Stroke

Someone suffers a **stroke** in the UK every five minutes (100,000 annually). The majority of strokes occur because clots in the circulation stop blood bringing oxygen to the brain. In most of these cases prompt attendance at hospital can lead to a clot-busting treatment that improves outcomes. Other strokes occur because of a bleed into the brain.

Symptoms are dependent on the location of the stroke but tend to come on rapidly. They include facial or limb weakness, slurred speech, visual impairment, confusion and dizziness or numbness.

Almost two thirds of stroke survivors leave hospital with a disability, often requiring significant support for the rest of their lives. One third of stroke victims experience depression afterwards.

Strokes are the fourth biggest killer in the UK, killing one person every thirteen seconds. Because of better recognition, quicker help-seeking and better treatments the death rate from stroke is half that of thirty years ago.

Support group:
Stroke Association (www.stroke.org.uk)

The Fall

The novel **SARS coronavirus-2** has already killed a million people worldwide, caused the worst global recession since the Great Depression of the 1930s and changed the way many of us live our daily lives. Last year it was the second-deadliest infectious disease worldwide, behind only tuberculosis for global mortality.

In Britain at least one in eight Covid-19 cases in hospital were contracted while there. Older age, male gender, south Asian ethnicity, obesity, poor cardiovascular health, lung disease and cancer put people at significantly greater risk of dying from the disease.

Bob

Dementia encompasses a range of diseases that cause a persistent decline in brain function – memory, language, problem-solving and other thinking skills – and affect a person's ability to perform everyday activities. As we live longer more of us are affected by the disease: 7% of over-sixty-fives have dementia, 17% of over-eighties and 40% of over-ninety-fives. In 2018 dementia became the leading cause of death in the UK for the first time.

The presentation of dementia in a person can vary wildly depending on their underlying brain function, the severity of the disease and the variability of the disease.

Another variable that affects the person with dementia is the environment around them. Tedium, inconsistency and change are all liable to increase anxiety and agitation. While the effects of dementia are often devastating on the sufferer and their loved ones, getting the right support is essential for better outcomes. Some researchers believe if we study, resource and tailor care around the illness sufficiently well we can turn it into a positive period of human life.

Support groups:
Dementia UK (www.dementiauk.org), Alzheimer's Society (www.alzheimers.org.uk); Age UK (www.ageuk.org.uk)

Bunker

Prostate cancer is the most common cancer suffered by men in the UK with 50,000 new diagnoses annually. It is increasingly common the older a man gets, and is most often diagnosed between the ages of seventy-five and seventy-nine years. It is usually slow-growing, and if caught early can often be treated successfully. In the 1970s only a quarter of men would survive ten years after their diagnosis; now that figure is 78%. Most men who have it will die of other causes. Nonetheless, it kills 12,000 men a year.

Screening for prostate cancer is not currently recommended, but men suffering from difficulties in passing urine should discuss this with their doctors as a simple examination and blood test can be helpful in working out who is at risk. Improved diagnosis probably accounts for the improvement in outcomes. If Clive had raised his concerns with doctors, he would have discovered quickly that there were alternative ways to image his prostate that would not trigger his claustrophobia.

Support group:
Prostate Cancer UK (www.prostatecanceruk.org)

Murmur

Heart valve disease affects 2.5% of the UK population. It is predominantly an illness of old age with a prevalence of over 10% among people aged seventy-five and older. Causes include infections, immune disease and structural defects.

Hearts have four valves, any of which can become narrowed (stenosis) or floppy (causing regurgitation); the effects of this can range from the trivial to the life-threatening, affecting the heart's ability to distribute blood around the body and leading to sudden death or heart failure. Symptoms include chest pain, fainting and breathlessness. Treatment used to require open-heart surgery, but these days procedures are often carried out via a blood vessel in the wrist or groin.

Support group:
British Heart Foundation (www.bhf.org.uk)

References

Papers

Anagnostou, K., and Turner, P. J. (2019), 'Myths, facts and controversies in the diagnosis and management of anaphylaxis', *Archives of Disease in Childhood*

Angst, J. et al (2016), 'The epidemiology of common mental disorders from age 20 to 50: results from the prospective Zurich cohort study', *Epidemiology and Psychiatric Sciences*

Brent, D. A. et al (1993), 'Psychiatric sequelae to the loss of an adolescent peer to suicide', *Journal of the American Academy of Child and Adolescent Psychiatry*

Christianson, A. et al (2006), 'Global report of birth defects: the hidden toll of dying and disabled', March of Dimes Birth Defects Foundation

Copeland, W. et al (2011), 'Cumulative prevalence of psychiatric disorders by young adulthood: a prospective cohort analysis from the Great Smoky Mountain Study', *Journal of the American Academy of Child and Adolescent Psychiatry*

Hasle, H. (2001), 'Pattern of malignant disorders in individuals with Down's syndrome', *Lancet Oncology*

Hawton, K., and Fagg, J. (1998), 'Suicide, and other causes of death, following attempted suicide', *British Journal of Psychiatry*

Jenkins, A., Millar, S., and Robins, J. (2011), 'Denial of pregnancy – a literature review and discussion of ethical and legal issues', *Journal of the Royal Society of Medicine*

Lawrence, T. et al (2016), 'Traumatic brain injury in England and Wales: prospective audit of epidemiology, complications and standardised mortality', *BMJ Open*

McAllister, T. W. (2008), 'Neurobehavioral sequelae of traumatic brain injury: evaluation and management', *World Psychiatry*

Nutt, D. (2020), 'New psychoactive substances: pharmacology influencing UK practice, policy and the law', *British Journal of Clinical Pharmacology*

Owens, D., Horrocks, J., and House, A. (2002), 'Fatal and non-fatal repetition of self-harm: systematic review', *British Journal of Psychiatry*

Ozturk, H. M. et al (2019), 'Synthetic cannabinoids and cardiac arrhythmia risk: review of the literature', *Cardiovascular Toxicology*.

Perkins, G. D. et al (2016), 'National initiatives to improve outcomes from out-of-hospital cardiac arrest in England', *Emergency Medicine Journal*

Rowland, T. A., and Marwaha, S. (2018), 'Epidemiology and risk factors for bipolar disorder', *Therapeutic Advances in Psychopharmacology*

Salavera, S., Tricás, J., and Lucha, O. et al (2011), 'Personality disorders and psychosocial problems in a group of participants to therapeutic processes for people with severe social disabilities', *BMC Psychiatry*

Schaefer, J. D. et al (2017), 'Enduring mental health: prevalence and prediction', *Journal of Abnormal Psychology*

Solevik, M. et al (2016), 'Visual Hallucinations used to be considered unlikely in First-Episode Psychosis: Association with Childhood Trauma', *PLOS One*

Spielvogel, A. M., Hohener, H. C. (1995), 'Denial of pregnancy: a review and case reports', *Birth*

Wessel, J., Gauruder-Burmester, A., and Gerlinger, C. (2007), 'Denial of pregnancy – characteristics of women at risk', *Acta Obstetricia Gynecologica Scandinavica*

Wissenberg, M. et al (2013), 'Association of national initiatives to improve cardiac arrest management with rates of bystander intervention and patient survival after out-of-hospital cardiac arrest', *JAMA*

Other Resources

British Heart Foundation Statistics Factsheet 2020

British Thyroid Foundation

Cancer Research UK

Centers for Disease Control and Prevention

Combat Stress, 'Reviewing the efficacy of case management for veterans with substance misuse problems', Ashwick, R. and Murphy, D.

Crime Survey of England and Wales 2018

Down's Syndrome Association

Euthanasia, NHS

Harvard Women's Health Watch

REFERENCES

Homeless Link, 'The unhealthy state of homelessness: health audit results 2014'

House of Commons Health and Social Care Committee, 'Prison Health, 2017–19'

House of Commons, Knife crime statistics

Institute for Health Metrics and Evaluation, 'Global Burden of Disease, 2017'

Mental Health of Children and Young People in England 2017, NHS digital

Mental Health Foundation

National Aids Trust

National Hip Fracture Database, 'Annual report 2017'

National Institutes of Health, Prader–Willi Syndrome

NICE Position Statement on Schizophrenia 2017

Nuffield Family Justice Observatory

Office for National Statistics, 'Statistics on alcohol, England 2018'

Office for National Statistics, 'Deaths of homeless people in England and Wales: 2013 to 2017'

'Protecting People Promoting Health: A public health approach to violence prevention for England, Department of Health, 2012', Department of Health and Social Care

'Resuscitation to recovery', Resuscitation Council, 2017

Tommy's

UNAIDS

Acknowledgements

Reuben Cohen and Louis Moulay-Mesiah whose passion for writing still propels me.

All of the amazing doctors who have taught me and guided me into medicine and those who helped and encouraged me to write this book.

My friend and super-agent Ellie Birne who made the book happen and shepherded it all the way through.

The magnificent Michael Joseph team, especially Rowland White, Ruth Atkins and Jennie Roman, for taking an idea and turning it into a book.

For vital technical assistance, Arun Menon, Andy Butterfield, Shigong Guo.

My astute and insightful readers, including Jai Amin, Chris Bird, Zachary Chan, Felicity Elwin, Alison Fairley, Asli Kalin, Ned Kelly, Lisa Miller, Richard Harrington, Dave Scott, Adam Smyth, Leelaa Templeton, Joseph Templeton and Siobhán Templeton.

The Templeton and Pattinson families, for their love and support.

Siobhán, Oscar, Molly and Sam, for their tolerance of my failings, their laughter and their love.